Breathe Slower, Deeper, Better

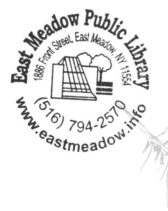

Breathe Slower, Deeper, Better

MAKE DEEP BREATHING A HABIT WITH SIMPLE YOGA EXERCISES

Yael Bloch

Illustrated by Cléo Werhlin

Translated by Julia Sanches

THE EXPERIMENT

NEW YORK

The Experiment, LLC
220 East 23rd Street, Suite 600
New York, NY 10010-4658
theexperimentpublishing.com

The Experiment's books are available at special discounts when purchased in bulk for premiums and sales promotions as well as for fund-raising or educational use. For details, contact us at info@theexperimentpublishing.com.

Library of Congress Cataloging-in-Publication Data

Names: Bloch, Yael, author.
Title: Breathe slower, deeper, better : make deep breathing a habit with simple yoga exercises / Yael Bloch ; illustrated by Cléo Werhlin ; translated by Julia Sanches.
Other titles: Respire. English
Description: New York : The Experiment, 2019.
Identifiers: LCCN 2019030649 (print) | LCCN 2019030650 (ebook) | ISBN 9781615195411 (trade paperback) | ISBN 9781615195992 (ebook)
Subjects: LCSH: Relaxation. | Meditation. | Yoga.
Classification: LCC RA785 .B5913 2017 (print) | LCC RA785 (ebook) | DDC 613/.192--dc23
LC record available at https://lccn.loc.gov/2019030649
LC ebook record available at https://lccn.loc.gov/2019030650

ISBN 978-1-61519-598-5
Ebook ISBN 978-1-61519-599-2

Cover and text design by Beth Bugler
Author photograph by Géraldine Borderie

Manufactured in China

First printing October 2019
10 9 8 7 6 5 4 3 2 1

We share breath,
breathing, and air with
the rest of humanity.
It takes us somewhere
extraordinary. We're alive
only because something
that can never be ours
courses through us.

—ISABELLE MORIN-LARBEY

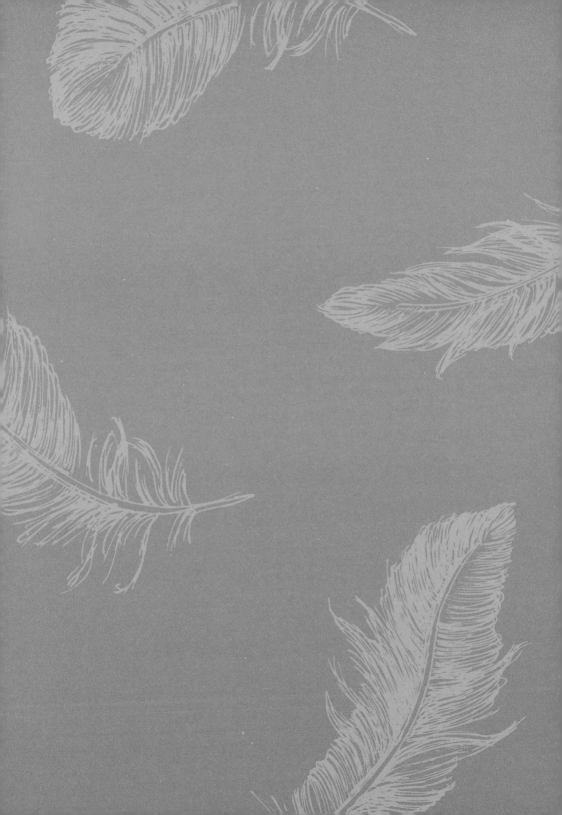

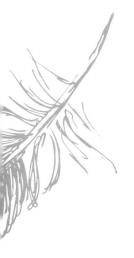

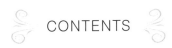 CONTENTS

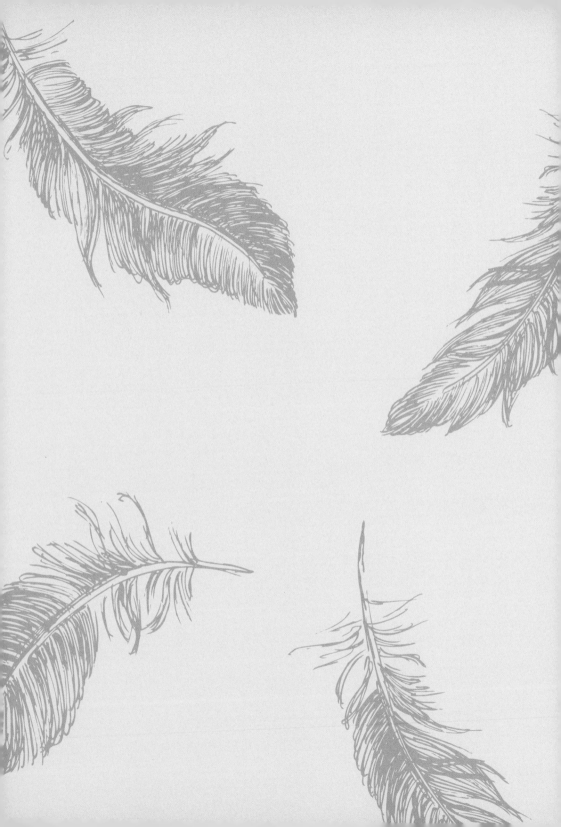

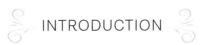

INTRODUCTION

I t's not unusual these days to hear someone tell a person who's stressed out to "Breathe!" Breathing is one of our most vital and basic processes. Because we do it without thinking, we tend to believe our bodies can breathe naturally. But there's breathing and then there's *breathing*. Natural breathing adapts itself to life's circumstances and, more often than not, has already been altered by factors tied to our past experience (education, stress, pollution, illness). We've developed breathing habits of varying efficiency, patterns we readily return to even while sleeping.

When we tell someone to breathe without any further instruction, they automatically and unconsciously breathe more deeply, but that's not necessarily the best or most appropriate response in a given situation.

That said, nothing is set in stone. According to one philosophy of yoga,* the same mechanisms that have cemented one habit can be used to forge another. This is our brains' capacity for what Western science refers to as "neuroplasticity," the brain's ability to reorganize itself by forming new neural connections over time.

---

* This is the theory of *samskaras*, which states that we have imprints that are left behind by habit that we resort to automatically.

What we need is to understand how breathing works, observe our breathing habits, and know that we can change them—or rather, reeducate them. Then we can determine whether they should be changed and, if need be, learn how to do so and then establish a practice to put in place. That is this book's main goal.

I've lived through this process myself. Having practiced yoga since the age of six and taught it since 2000, I thought I knew how to breathe. You can imagine my surprise, then, when I was informed by a hypnotist, a speech-language pathologist, and a singing teacher that I was breathing incorrectly. These professionals each dealt me an irrevocable diagnosis without any explanation, or at least not one I truly understood. I was left with a huge question mark. The only thing I knew was that something had to change. But what?

For years, this question remained unsolved. Whenever I heard or read anything about breathing, my whole body became alert, focused on unraveling this mystery to reach beyond what I might read or hear and produce the spark of understanding that had been eluding me. This understanding eventually came to me not as a revelation but as a certainty that, little by little, settled into my body, became a conscious thought, and then was able to be expressed.

But the motivating factor for this book was something I witnessed in 2017. I used to believe that, while sleeping, we systematically fell into a balanced abdominal breathing. But I received resounding proof to the contrary when, at the close of a yoga class that ended in a deep relaxation, one of the practitioners fell asleep and began to breathe slowly, strongly, and deeply. The rise and fall of the woman's belly and chest was highly visible and I could tell she was breathing "backward"—when she inhaled, her chest contracted, and when she exhaled, her chest expanded. This was the moment I understood that, when we're faced with deep-set bad breathing habits, finding our proper breath requires more than a relaxed mind and body. And if bad habits persist under conditions of optimal relaxation—a deep sleep, for example—they're obviously also present when we're awake.

Yoga practitioners will recognize certain basic traditional teachings throughout the book. Two doctors, Guy Taïeb and Andrée Maman, and one osteopath, Jean-Pierre Laffez, with whom I had the opportunity of working and speaking, were immensely helpful to me in shaping this book. All three of them are also wonderful yoga instructors.

To begin, there are two tests that will help you identify some of your automatisms as you read this book. The chapters that follow will serve as a recap of our breathing mechanisms and the muscles involved. Then, the book will lay the foundations for how we should breathe while lying down, before going on to outline the sorts of poor breathing habits we sometimes fall into. It will focus on the interplay between breathing and position and movement, on the one hand, and emotion on the other. The final chapter will guide you through a simple and accessible practice, inspired in large part by yoga, to implement good breathing habits that will be beneficial for your health and wellness.

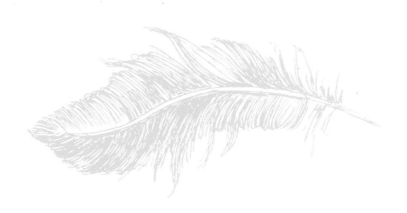

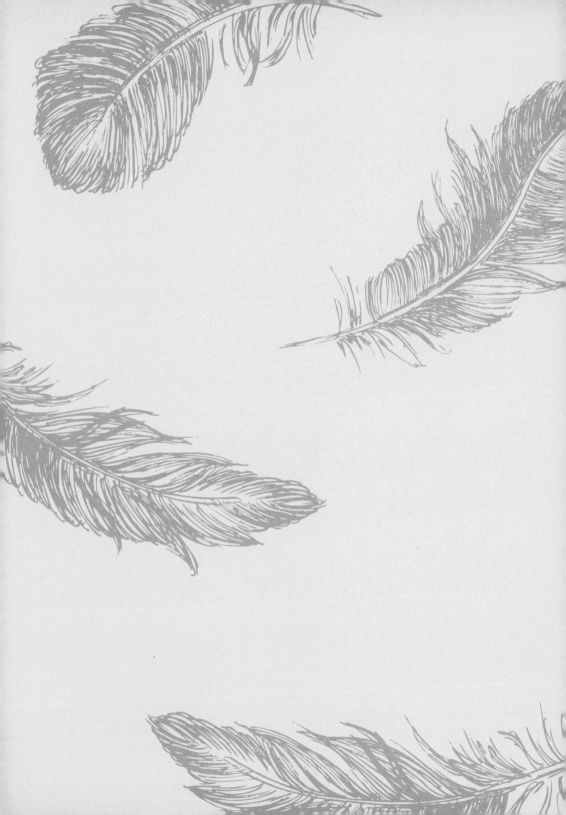

CHAPTER 1

Identify Your Breathing Habits

The following tests can be completed at any time. That said, if you're able to do them before reading the following chapters, they'll help you access valuable information about your regular, automatic breathing habits, as well as the way your pelvic floor works. When you are in the standing position, your pelvic floor forms a sling from the coccyx and the sacrum, in the back, to the pubis, in the front. This muscle holds the viscera of the pelvic cavity, and you can feel its surface layer tensing at skin level.* You may be asking yourself what the pelvic floor is doing in a book about breathing, but you'll find out soon enough.

If you read the rest of the book first, you may find your attitude unconsciously changed when you take these tests, and the results might not account for your usual automatisms. Don't try to figure out or picture what you think you should do. Instead, try to be as spontaneous as possible. You'll learn a lot more about yourself this way.

* The internal surface sensation must be distinguished from more localized sensations around this area's sphincters (the anus, the urethra, and the vagina), which are circular muscles that contract reflexively.

Test 1

MATERIALS

Measuring tape, chair.

The following can be done on your own or, better yet, with someone to help take measurements, allowing you to remain still and focused on your usual breathing.

IN THE LYING POSITION

Begin in a relaxed position, with your legs extended.

Wrap the tape measure around your waist. Measure once at the end of your inhalation and again at the end of your exhalation, then enter these measurements into the table below. Take these measurements again, this time around your underwear band: The tape measure should pass slightly to the right of your iliac crest (lower waist). The idea is to have a clear marker so that you can measure around the same place in both positions. What happens as you inhale and exhale? Is your belly moving, or not? What direction is it moving in? When does it deflate, and when does it inflate? Record the answers to these questions.

IN THE SEATED POSITION

Repeat the measurements above while sitting comfortably in a chair. Your spine should be erect, without touching the chair back. Take measurements at waist height, then around your lower waist, and jot down the information. Ask yourself the questions listed in the previous paragraph and record.

MEASUREMENT CHART

MEASUREMENT		LYING POSITION	SEATED POSITION
Waist	Inhaling		
	Exhaling		
Lower waist	Inhaling		
	Exhaling		

Test results are decoded in chapters 4 and 6.

Breathe Slower, Deeper, Better

Test 2

MATERIALS

Large pillow, blanket (optional).

EXERCISE

Kneel, straddling the pillow *(image 1)*. If the floor is too hard, place a blanket or pillow beneath your knees. If the pressure on your knees is too intense and you experience pain, add another pillow or blanket. Find a comfortable position. The surface muscles of your pelvic floor should be in direct contact with the pillow.

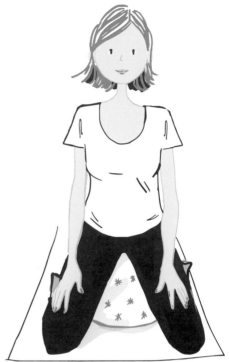

Image 1

- Pretend to blow up a balloon. If you happen to have one on hand, you can actually use it. Pay attention to the sensations around your pelvic floor. Does contact with the pillow make these sensations intensify or diminish, or do they stay the same?

- Now, pretend to cough. Once again, note the sensations around your pelvic floor.

- Record your observations.

Test results are decoded in chapter 4.

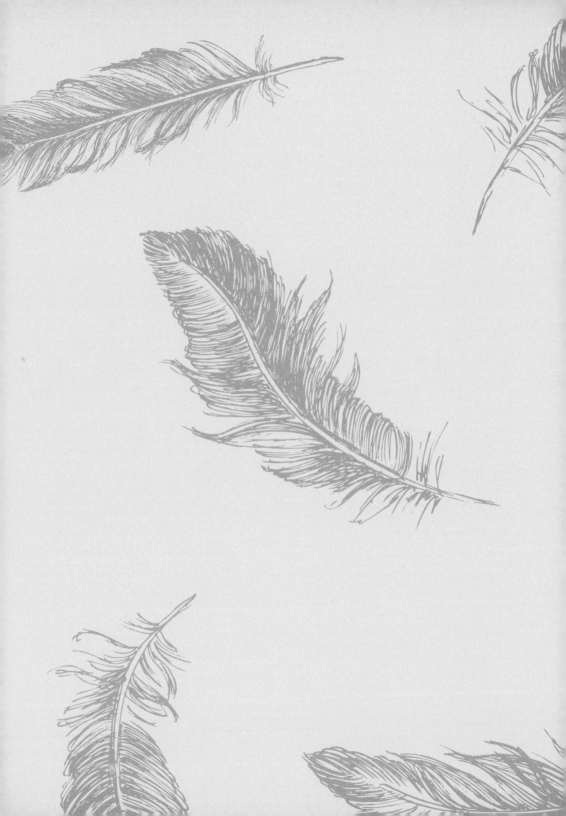

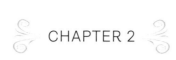

CHAPTER 2

How to Breathe

In this book, most of our focus will be on the torso. But when it comes to taking in air, should we be breathing through our nose or our mouth? Or does it even matter?

When you run, your breathing accelerates and you're forced to breathe through your mouth, allowing for faster external gas exchange, during both inhalation and exhalation. But physiological breathing is nasal—newborns breathe almost exclusively through their noses. Mouth breathing is seen as "rescue" breathing, with a few exceptions: sighing, coughing, blowing out air, whistling, speaking, and singing all occur through the mouth. In yoga, there is mantra recitation or singing, cooling breathing (in which you inhale through the mouth and exhale through the nose) and cleansing breathing (in which you only exhale through the mouth). But breathing should mostly occur through the nose.

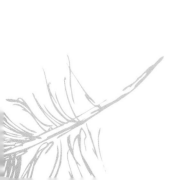
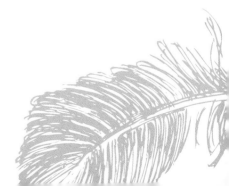

WHY DOES MOST BREATHING HAPPEN THROUGH THE NOSE IN YOGA?

- Nose breathing slows down both inhalation and exhalation because the distance traveled is greater from the nose than it is from the mouth. In the exercises in which our breath alternates (each nostril closed by turns), or during throat-holding (*ujjayi pranayama; see page 66*), the constriction of airways is accentuated, triggering a lull.

- When breathing through the nose, air passes various cavities, or folds, called "conchae," which extend the mucous surface and make it more efficient at heating up the air to the body's temperature and achieving the right humidity.

- This is best perceived as the air enters the nostrils, which is much more noticeable during inhalation than exhalation because the inhaled air is at a cooler temperature than the body. You can test the humidity and warmth of the exhaled air by placing your finger a couple of millimeters beneath your nostrils.*

- Nasal mucosa also plays an antibacterial role.[1]

- The nose also serves as a filter. Nasal buildup is a good indicator of how contaminated or pure the air is. This filtering happens during inhalation. But if you always inhale through your nose and exhale through your mouth, your nose will become dry—because the air inhaled is drier than the body. In yoga, breathing is done principally through the nose in order to maintain a balanced level of moisture in the nose.

---

* To encounter more precise sensations around the nostrils, *anapana* (as taught in Vipassana meditation techniques) can be of great interest.

Breathe Slower, Deeper, Better

- The nostrils are the points of entrance for the two energy channels, the nadis *ida* and *pingala,* and all breathing exercises that alternately engage the nostrils will promote balance between these two channels and, more generally, between the pairs of opposites within us, especially on the energetic level.

WHEN PASSING THE NASAL MUCOSA, THE AIR TOUCHES A MULTITUDE OF SENSORY RECEPTORS. THESE SEND OFF INFORMATION TO THE BRAIN AND ENERGY CIRCUITS. BY LEARNING TO MANIPULATE AIR WHEN IT TOUCHES THE MUCOSA, THE YOGI CAN REGULATE THE BODY'S MECHANISMS.[2]

Nasal breathing isn't always possible, either on a temporary basis, due to a cold, for example, or a permanent one, due to an illness or after an accident. In these cases, breathing occurs through the mouth. In cases of deviated nasal septa, for example, when there is respiratory asymmetry between both nostrils, the alternating breathing exercises in this book will have to be adapted.[*]

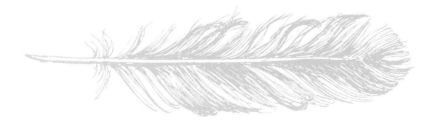

---

[*] In these cases, Yoga de l'Énergie puts forward an energetic framework that can impact both energy channels, even when mouth breathing in alternation.

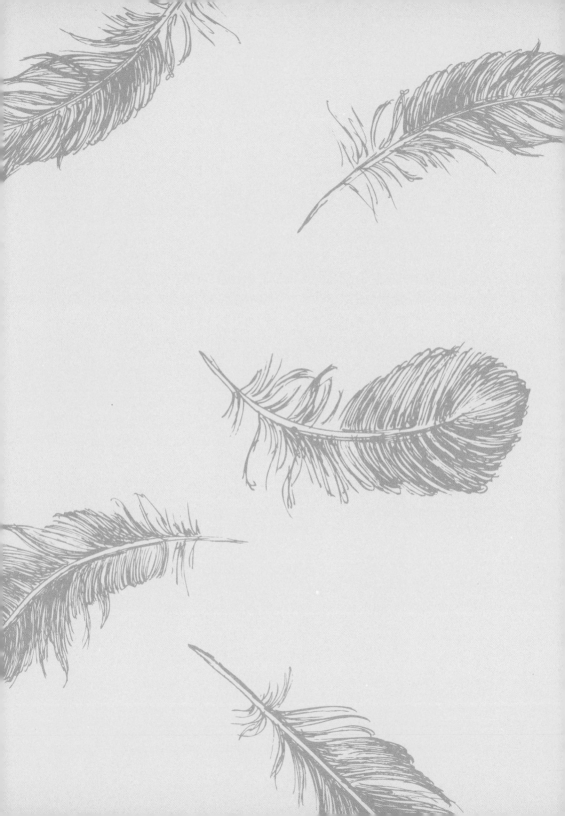

CHAPTER 3

The Mechanics of Breathing

According to Western science—though this is also the case in Indian tradition—**breathing's primary function is to obtain energy**. Strictly speaking, breathing involves four processes:

1. **External respiration, or pulmonary ventilation,** between our lungs and the air outside.

2. **External gas exchange**, which takes place at the intersection between the lungs' alveoli and capillaries.

3. **Transportation,** in which the entire bloodstream—even the smallest vessels—carries oxygen (O_2) to the approximately 60,000 billion cells throughout the body—to muscles, organs, and tissues.

4. **Cellular respiration,** the cornerstone of the entire process: "Food and O_2 molecules are both turned into exploitable energy for our cells."[3] This transformation takes place constantly. Though indispensable to the process, oxygen cannot be stored in our cells, which means we need a constant supply of it. Our cells discard carbon dioxide in exchange for oxygen—this is the eliminatory function of breathing *(image 2)*. After our

cells produce CO_2, the blood immediately carries it to the lungs for us to breathe out.

This book only covers pulmonary ventilation, more commonly referred to as breathing. I will occasionally use this term throughout.

Image 2

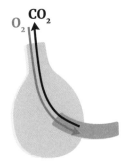

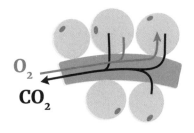

External gas exchange

Gas exchange between cells and blood

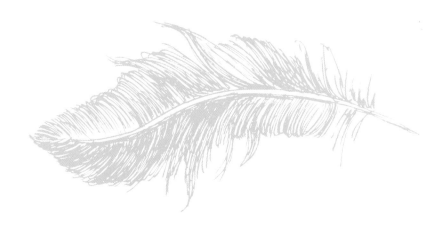

Image 3

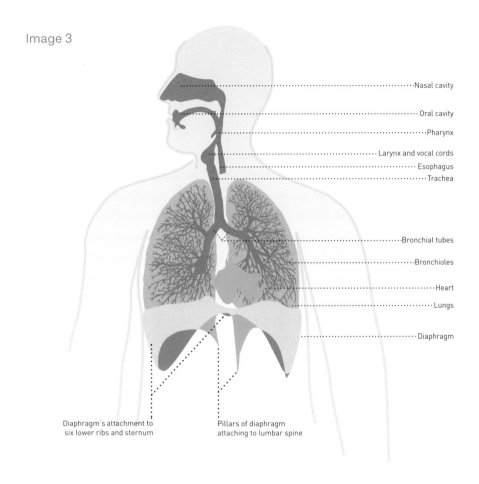

Nasal cavity

Oral cavity

Pharynx

Larynx and vocal cords

Esophagus

Trachea

Bronchial tubes

Bronchioles

Heart

Lungs

Diaphragm

Diaphragm's attachment to
six lower ribs and sternum

Pillars of diaphragm
attaching to lumbar spine

Image 4

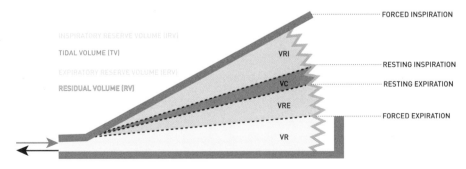

INSPIRATORY RESERVE VOLUME (IRV)

TIDAL VOLUME (TV)

EXPIRATORY RESERVE VOLUME (ERV)

RESIDUAL VOLUME (RV)

FORCED INSPIRATION

VRI

RESTING INSPIRATION

VC

RESTING EXPIRATION

VRE

FORCED EXPIRATION

VR

Anatomy

Our respiratory system (*image 3*) is made up of the nose, pharynx, larynx, trachea, and two lungs, right and left, each with its own right primary bronchus, which branches into bronchiole, in turn ending in pulmonary alveoli, 300 million tiny pockets that fill with air, then empty. If expanded, their surface area would be around 200 square feet (60 square meters).

This is the site of the gas exchange: The air in the alveoli is oxygen rich—at 21 percent—and the blood enters the lungs heavy with the cells' discarded carbon dioxide. At the end of the gas exchange, there is an equal concentration of each—O_2 and CO_2—in the blood and in the air. In other words, the blood loses carbon dioxide and becomes rich in oxygen, and vice versa for exhaled air, whose O_2 concentration remains at 17 percent. I love Guy Taïeb's comment on this process: "This is the only example of an encounter between rich and poor in which, when both leave, one is just as rich as the other. The rich one doesn't become any poorer, because the more it gives, the more it gets!"[4]

The respiratory control center, in the brain stem, is sensitive to the most minute variations in O_2 and CO_2 pressure and concentration in the blood. It seeks to maintain this consistency by automatically adjusting our breathing rhythms to different circumstances. For example, an increase in CO_2 pressure will often trigger inhalation.

The Mechanics of Ventilation

In the West, "breathing," or pulmonary ventilation, is divided into two phases: inhalation and exhalation.

We tend to think our lungs fill *because* we take a breath of air. But it's actually the opposite. When the body needs oxygen, our medulla oblongata, located beneath the brain, evaluates the situation and sends a nerve impulse to the inspiratory muscles (see chapter 4). When these muscles contract, our rib cage and lungs expand, creating an indraft: hence, inhalation, air filling the lungs. Seeing that the need for oxygen has been met, the medulla oblongata stops stimulating the inspiratory muscles, resulting in exhalation, air expelled from the lungs.

Respiratory Volumes

The volume of air we use while resting, known as the tidal volume (TV), is around 0.13 gallons (0.5 liters). This figure corresponds to a statistical average and does not take into account variations in age, sex, morphology, or individual respiratory training. For this reason, it should not be taken as an ideal value but rather a reflection of our strict breathing habits, and this statistical average is lower than it would be if everyone breathed properly. But anyone can use breathing techniques to increase their tidal volume.

When we are breathing "deeply," our respiratory volume is higher. This volume varies from person to person, but it can also be improved with training *(image 4)*.

- The inspiratory reserve volume (IRV) is the maximum volume that a person can inhale outside their resting breath, and ranges from 0.5 to 0.8 gallons (2 to 3 liters) of air.

- The expiratory reserve volume (ERV) is the maximum volume that a person can exhale outside their resting breath, ranging from 0.25 to 0.4 gallons (1 to 1.5 liters) of air. At the end of an ERV exhalation, the lungs empty, though never entirely: A certain volume of air always remains, around 0.4 gallons (1.5 liters), known as the residual volume (RV). Stirred by ventilation, this air ensures the continuation of the alveolar-capillary exchange.

The Yogic Perspective

Breathing is the only involuntary (automatic and unconscious) function that can be willfully modified, hence yogis' age-old interest in it.

The ancient Upanishads, written between 800 BCE and 500 BCE, illustrate India's fascination with this vital and mysterious force known as *prana*, which fills us and leaves us. The Upanishads illustrate the supremacy of breath over the body's other faculties—the mind, speech, hearing, and sight—which are personified in the text. In a dispute over their superiority, each entity leaves the body, one by one, without impairing any of the body's essential functions. But when the prana begins to leave, and the body starts to die, the other entities become aware of its superiority and plead for its return.*

Prana is much more than air. And breathing is not just a matter of gas exchanges or the physical functions mentioned earlier. It affects everything on the energetic, mental, emotional, and spiritual levels. The prana occupies a central place, which has been described in several Upanishads with help from the following metaphor: "As spokes in the nave of a wheel, everything is fixed in the prana."† It is prana that sustains every manifestation of life, movement, and energy; prana that expresses itself in gravitational, electric, and magnetic forces, and also in our body's inner movements.

- *Prana* means "energy that anchors the living," vital energy (the root *an* can be found in the Latin word *anima* and in the French word for soul, *âme*).

- *Yama* means to subdue, tame, keep on a leash (the idea being of control).

---

* For example: *Prashna Upanishad* (II, 1–4), *Chandogya Upanishad* (V, I, I, 1–5), *Brihadaranyaka Upanishad* (VI, I, 1–14).

† *Prashna Upanishad* (II, 6).

By combining both we get "pranayama": a form of breathing (in terms of the physical, rhythmic, durational, respiratory gymnastics).

The word can also be broken down as *prana-ayama*: the art of breathing (in terms of the subtlety of breath, awareness without altering its mechanism).

These two definitions are complementary and together refer to the practice of pranayama.

Though pranayama occurs in the physical body, it resonates on other levels. When breathing is expansive and refined, it becomes breath. By attending to breath, which enters and leaves us, we are met with a vibrant presence, a sense of being in permanent dialogue with the world around us, and a feeling of deep gratitude—because without breath there is no life.

The Upanishads also explain that prana is divided into five breaths[*] with the following complementary functions: assimilation, elimination, communication with the exterior, balance, and diffusion.

In yoga, breathing occurs in four stages. These include inhalation, full-lung suspension of breath after inhalation, exhalation, and an empty-lung suspension[†] of breath after exhalation. *The Yoga-Sutra of Patañjali,* which dates to sometime between 200 BCE and 200 CE, is a record of practices of that time (II, 50): "Pranayama manifests as external, internal, and restrained movements [of breath]."[5] Naming these breathing stages allowed for the development of yogic breathwork.

Good oxygenation and good breathing are essential for our body to work at its best and for us to remain in good health.

An important point: Contrary to popular belief, which would lead us to think we need oxygen most of all during physical exertion, **we actually need oxygen just as much when resting, simply for thinking.** The brain takes up

---

[*] For example: *Prashna Upanishad* (III, 1–9), *Taittiriya Upanishad* (I, VII, 1).

[†] We speak of "apnea" in medical terms, while in yoga, the term used is "retention" and, more uncommonly, "blockage." I prefer "suspension," which influences our lived practice, making it, to my mind, softer, finer, truer.

20 percent of the body's overall oxygen use, so actively learning to breathe is fundamental. Only after doing so can we achieve our lungs' optimal condition, with all the alveoli playing the role nature intended to their full capacity.

How we breathe can have a significant impact on every aspect of our lives. Not only does it influence the way we think and focus, it also affects our respiratory, cardiovascular, neurological, gastrointestinal, muscular, immunological, hormonal, psychological, and psychosomatic systems, and impacts our stress endurance, quality of sleep, memory, aging, ability to stop and unwind, and our energy levels and worldview.

In chapter 4, we will, above all, look at ways of breathing. It's worth remembering that breathing also depends in part on the verticality and suppleness of the spinal cord and the flexibility of the thorax. It's worth working on these separately, too.

Breathe Slower, Deeper, Better

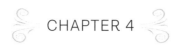

CHAPTER 4

Respiratory Muscles

Breathing at Rest

Our resting breath activates our primary respiratory muscles—the diaphragm and the intercostal muscles—as well as the lower rib cage. In fact, the lower rib cage is where breathing is at its most effective because this is the widest part of the torso and the breadth of movement is optimal, since the floating ribs aren't attached to the sternum.

The diaphragm is an astonishing muscle, responsible for 75 percent of our respiratory efforts.[6] Shaped like a dome, it splits the torso into two parts—the thorax and the abdomen. Crossed by the esophagus and the aorta, the diaphragm is a muscular crown with a white, fibrous center known as the central tendon. It is attached to the sternum and six lower ribs, as well as the inner surface of the lumbar spine via inserts (image 3). Because it has very few sensory receptors, we can't usually feel the diaphragm contracting.

NATIVE AMERICANS SAW THE DIAPHRAGM AS THE HORIZON BETWEEN HEAVEN AND EARTH.[7]

Inhalation results from the contraction of the diaphragm and external intercostal muscles. The diaphragm lowers, then flattens. Supported by the viscera, it triggers the expansion and elevation of the lower ribs in a "bucket handle" motion. The chest swells, especially near the lower diaphragm. The belly thrusts downward, deforming and swelling simultaneously.

Inhalation is a muscular exertion; it is the active phase of breath. Each inhalation is a life-giving effort. It's impossible not to be buoyed by the thought that we accomplish this feat after each exhalation, approximately 21,600 times a day—an average of 15 breaths per minute—day after day.

While exhaling, our rib cage and lungs retract elastically.* The diaphragm once again relaxes and rises. This is followed by the equally elastic return of the abdominal muscles, which extend during inhalation. Both belly and chest settle *(image 5)*. The resting position of the lungs and rib cage is marked by the end of the exhalation.

Exhalation is a muscular relaxation; it is the passive, gentle breathing phase.

Naturally, our very first respiratory movement at birth is inhalation. This is an essential action that allows the newborn to shift from fetal-placental oxygenation to pulmonary oxygenation with the expansion of the lung's alveoli. Our very first inhalation remains a mystery "moved by an energy

---

* You'll find the concept of "pulmonary elasticity," or *élastique pulmonaire,* in Blandine Calais-Germain's book *Respiration, anatomie, geste respiratoire.*

Image 5

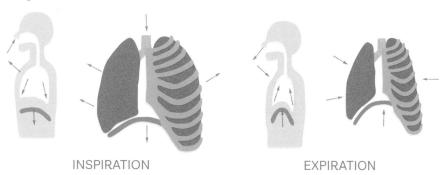

INSPIRATION   EXPIRATION

that existed before that moment,"[8] writes Jean-Pierre Laffez. And our lives end with a final exhalation—we often speak of taking "our last breath."

Not only is the diaphragm's movement crucial to breathing, but it also plays an important role in massaging our organs and viscera—essential for abdominal peristalsis—and in massaging the heart, located directly above it. It also stimulates the circulatory and lymphatic systems.[9] The broader the movement of the diaphragm, the more "all these organs are massaged, rolled, churned, bathed in new blood, fluids, and oxygen. [As the diaphragm moves,] the organs get squeezed and released like sponges."[10]

Deep Breathing*

Although deep breathing engages the same muscles cited above, it extends beyond the tidal volume, actively mobilizing our secondary respiratory muscles, especially the abdominal muscles, the pectoralis major and minor, the sternocleidomastoid, and the scalene (neck muscles).[†]

---

* "Deep" and "long" are yogic terms; the medical term is "forced."

† Other muscles participate in this kind of breathing. For a more in-depth perspective, see Calais-Germain's *Respiration, anatomie, geste respiratoire*, which includes illustrated explanations on how to find each of our muscles based on the body's position and/or hand placement.

In a **deep inhalation** that follows a regular inhalation (at tidal volume), the volume of the rib cage, and therefore of the lungs, expands in every direction. The movement—previously centered on the lower ribs—now engages the entire thorax, all the way up to the first ribs (right beneath the clavicle). The sternum rises as the pectoral and neck muscles contract. This often creates the illusion that inhalation is an upward motion.

For the thorax to deform in this way, the central tendon, once it is at its lowest position, must be supported by the abdomen. An effective deep inhalation affects the full volume of the torso, all the way to the pelvic floor,[*] which bows slightly downward.[†]

Because of the contraction of our abdomen, a **deep exhalation** will exceed the tidal volume. Our abdominal volume is pushed either up or down, in a motion similar to squeezing a balloon with your hand *(images 6a and 6b)*. We know that an upward push follows the diaphragm's rise and facilitates exhalation. A downward push, toward the pelvic floor, which is a far more direct application of pressure than that applied to our diaphragm during inhalation, can be detrimental, even more so when applied brusquely, deeply, and repeatedly (such as when we laugh, sneeze, or cough). This affects the elasticity of the pelvic floor, which, if weakened, can lead to urine leakage, incontinence, or even organ prolapse.

To avoid these problems, we must tone the pelvic floor. This will protect and restore the diaphragm's respiratory synergy; the downward push spurred by abdominal contraction becomes an upward push, facilitating the

---

[*] In common parlance, "perineum" and "pelvic floor," and in some instances, "pelvic diaphragm," are used to designate the muscles that support the viscera of the pelvic cavity. Only specialists in this area draw a distinction between the two surface muscle layers (the perineum) and the deeper layer (the pelvic floor).

[†] In *The Breathing Book: Good Health and Vitality Through Essential Breath Work*, Donna Farhi notes that the same phenomenon can be seen around the vocal cords, which she refers to as the "vocal diaphragm," where relaxation, which corresponds to a lifting motion, promotes air intake during inhalation.

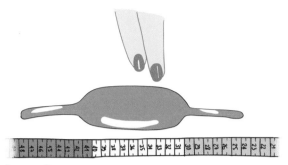

Image 6a

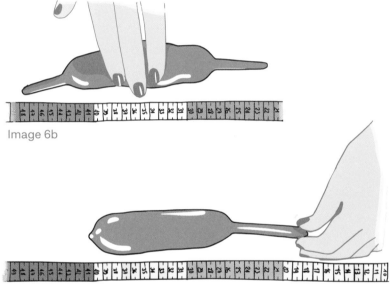

Image 6b

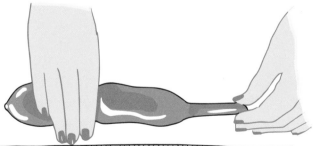

Image 6c

Image 6d

rise of the abdomen and, therefore, the diaphragm. In men, this can have substantial positive effects for the prevention or attenuation of prostate-related issues and the incontinence that often accompanies them. For every gender, toning the pelvic floor can also contribute to a vibrant sexual life.

Let's use our balloon again to illustrate this mechanism. By holding it tight and preventing it from moving down *(images 6c and 6d),* the pelvic floor muscles can only be angled upward. The goal of Test 2 in chapter 2 was to highlight your pelvic floor's spontaneous behavior under two different conditions. The first part examined its reaction to applied pressure, and the second took speed into account. You should have been able to make different observations from each of these tests.

If sensations around the point of contact with the pillow did not intensify, this means your pelvic floor remains engaged in every circumstance. If this is the case, it would be helpful to determine if it is permanently tensed, if you're able to relax it, and if you can tell the difference between several different degrees of contraction.

If you did feel the pressure of the pillow, your pelvic floor will have to be strengthened. You can practice doing the exercises again by contracting your pelvic floor. The exercise "Exhalation Work with Pelvic Floor," in chapter 9, will teach you how to gently tone this muscle and get it to work in sync with your breath. You might also consider seeking rehabilitation with a therapist.

WHY DO PEOPLE NEED TO GO TO THE BATHROOM DURING OR AFTER YOGA?[11]

Because deep breathing makes you want to pee! When the diaphragm moves, it massages the kidneys, which are located around the twelfth thoracic vertebra.

Breathe Slower, Deeper, Better

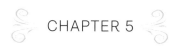
The Three Stages

Foundations for Good Breathing

In yoga, there are three separate breathing stages: abdominal breathing, which gets its name from the movement of our bellies; thoracic breathing; and chest, or clavicular, breathing.

When these three stages are engaged and in sync with our breath, the lungs are fulfilling their natural role, and the body is properly oxygenated. This is one facet of wellness. Our breathing is, at its most optimal, naturally expansive.

The best way to feel these three stages is on your back. It's easiest to focus clearly on breathing when the body is relaxed.

Lie on Your Back

Choose a hard but comfortable base (a yoga mat, if you have one). With your back on the floor, bring your knees up to your chest and rock side to side while softly stretching the back of your neck. Your chin should be slightly tucked—this will enable your body to settle into the floor gradually and allow you to feel your entire back touching the floor as your lumbar and cervical spine stretches. Next, extend your legs, one at a time. Place one shoulder on the ground, then the other, lifting and then lowering the shoulder blade toward the lower back. The shoulders should disengage from the head.

VARIATION

If you are uncomfortable and the back of your neck is too arched, place a small cushion beneath your head. But if possible, try not to use one.

In cases of lower back pain, place a cushion beneath your knees, or keep your knees bent and your feet on the ground, near the pelvic floor.

If this is too hard on your back, try placing your back against a sloped surface.

Observing Your Spontaneous Breath

Enter relaxation. "One way to do this is to use your mind and senses to follow the air's path through your body as it brushes past your naval cavity, your pharynx, your larynx, your trachea, bordering the front of your spine and filling your lungs, which are pressed against your diaphragm, which in turn pushes back your viscera. . . . Air flows unrestricted."[12]

Now, focus on your breath, with one hand on your belly and the other on your chest (image 7). Try to breathe normally. Where is your breath located, overall? Around your belly, your chest, or both? Is it regular, noisy, or fluid? Does it have naturally occurring suspensions? Which breathing phase do you enjoy the most? You can even count how many breaths you take per minute, and the length of each inhalation and exhalation.

Observing our "animal breath," as Roger Clerc calls it, "is a foundational exercise. We should do it as often as we can" because "it improves our concentration and soothes our minds."[13]

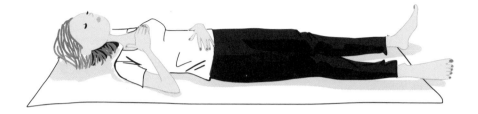

Becoming Aware of the Three Stages of Breathing

Your breath should be calm and easy. Spend a few breaths in each of the positions described below, centering your attention on your sensations, particularly beneath your hands. Next, stimulate your breath around the area in question by gently pushing down with your hands as you exhale. Then, release the pressure and, while inhaling, feel your body as it softly presses into your hands.

You can highlight each movement by breathing more loudly for a few breaths. To better mark your exhalation, try blowing out through your half-open mouth or making a noise.

> When we exhale through the mouth, the abdominal muscles are automatically engaged and the vocal cords draw closer, naturally giving way to a deeper and longer exhalation that's easier to perceive. Such is the case when we speak, sing, gasp, yawn, or sigh.

First Position: Abdominal Breathing

Place your hands on your belly so that the tips of your middle fingers touch as you exhale *(image 8a)*. This will make it easier to spot your hands drifting apart as you inhale, thus marking the rise of your belly *(image 8b)*. This is called "baby's breath," because it is highly visible in babies. Humans should be able to breathe well at the beginning of their lives. In some cases, it's also possible for a newborn's breathing to have been affected by jolts experienced during the mother's pregnancy.[14] Even so, the baby, unable to breathe air, "tries to overcome these different patterns by contracting the diaphragm . . . which sends soothing 'oxygen-full breaths' into its system."[15]

Recall the same sensations you experienced during Test 1 in chapter 2, in the lying position. If you were breathing paradoxically, or backward, the measurements taken will indicate that your belly deflated during inhalation and rose during exhalation. Try to reverse this habit. This process can take time, so don't worry if you don't manage it immediately. The mere awareness that it is possible to improve your breathing is already a big step, so be patient. Think about it when you get into bed, before you fall asleep. Picture a balloon that inflates during inhalation and deflates during exhalation. Remember, even though the goal is to develop a belly-focused movement, the point isn't to puff up your belly like a balloon either!

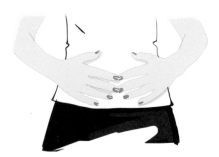

Image 8a

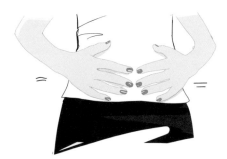

Image 8b

Second Position: Thoracic Breathing

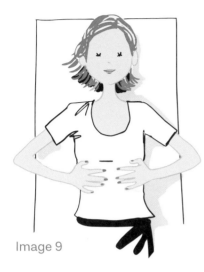

Image 9

Place your hands on your rib cage *(image 9),* level with your lower ribs. This way, you'll see your breath moving in every direction. Rear breathing is far less noticeable in this position, since you're limited by the back's contact with the floor. But think of dancers for a moment, and you'll see that this is how they breathe: Their abdominal muscles, usually contracted when in action, constrain their ability to breathe with their bellies, and their chest breathing is constrained by their attempt to hide their accelerated breath. But, look at their sides and you'll see the effects of their movements and leaps, their breath's exertion.

If you can't feel your lower ribs moving—as is often the case with people who are predominantly chest breathers—gently apply downward pressure on your ribs while exhaling, as if trying to get your right and left ribs to meet. Then, relax this pressure when inhaling and try to feel your ribs expanding as they push your hands up and to the side. Picture an accordion that opens during inhalation and closes during exhalation.

Third Position: Clavicular Breathing

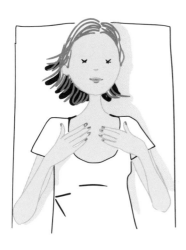

Image 10

Place your hands on your clavicles. Clavicular breathing is beneficial when used in addition to the two previous breathing stages and can be felt by setting your hands in this position. Picture a drawer that pulls out toward your chin when you inhale and closes when you exhale.

If you can only find your breath in this one spot, that's a sign of stress. This type of breathing requires a lot of effort for mediocre results. The shoulders lift so that only a small section of the lungs can fill to the max. Only a small percentage of our thoracic capacity is used.

Full Breathing with Arms*

This breathing method combines the three stages of inhalation and exhalation and ensures broad movement of the diaphragm and rib cage. "This broad respiratory movement makes room for new sensations that give new life to certain parts of the body,"[16] says Marie-Christine Leccia.

During inhalation, the diaphragm drops, pressing down on the abdomen, which lifts (abdominal breathing). Then, as the diaphragm meets resistance, the ribs open, all the way up the rib cage (thoracic and clavicular breathing). Follow this movement with your arms by spreading them open on the floor and sweeping them upward to the back of your head, like a child making a snow angel *(images 11a to 11d)*. The arms should extend, naturally triggering a suspension of breath and provoking a yawn or sigh.

* This movement is regularly practiced between positions at the École Française de Yoga.

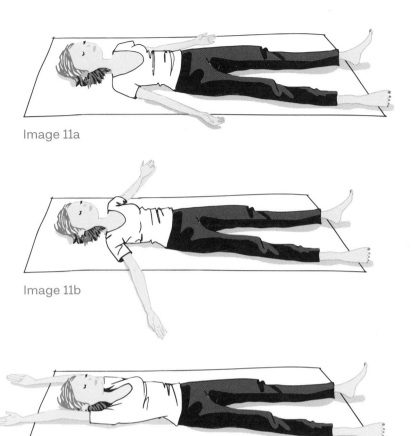

Image 11a

Image 11b

Image 11c

As you exhale, return your arms to the front, marking the end of the thoracic and abdominal stages.

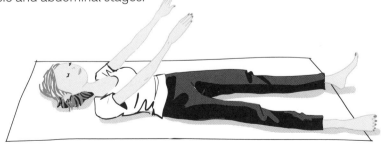

Image 11d

WE KNOW THAT BROAD RESPIRATORY MOVEMENTS
TRIGGER THE SECRETION OF ENDORPHINS, PLEASURE'S
NEUROMEDIATORS. SO WE CAN BETTER UNDERSTAND WHY
YOGA, WHICH PUTS BREATHING AT THE HEART OF ITS PRACTICE
BY PROMOTING A SUBTLE AND HIGH-QUALITY FULL BREATH, IS
SUCH A VITAL CONTRIBUTION TO WELLNESS!
—GUY TAÏEB

To try these breaths in the sitting or standing position, consult chapter 7 for variations.

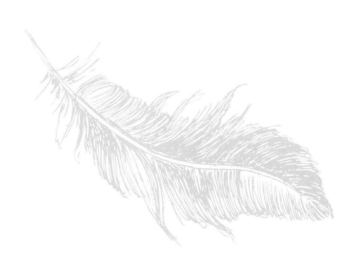

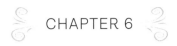

CHAPTER 6

Breathing
A Matter of Habit

Our breath constantly adapts to shifting circumstances and, over time, we've come to unconsciously develop certain routine breathing patterns. Habits become ingrained through repetition, and breathing is the gesture we repeat the most—approximately 21,600 times a day. Our breathing patterns are therefore deeply ingrained. Still—and this is one of yoga's pledges—we are not prisoners to our habits, everything can be transformed, and every breath is an opportunity to breathe differently, if we so desire. By relearning how to breathe, we can reprogram ourselves, becoming healthier in the process.*

There are many different forms of breathing, all with their advantages and disadvantages,† but certain forms should be avoided when in regular breathing positions (either seated or standing). Donna Farhi has identified seven ways of "breathing poorly"‡ and the effects they have on our minds and bodies.[17]

---

* Donna Farhi's *The Breathing Book* cites research that demonstrates the many things breathwork can improve, such as migraines.

† This is what Blandine Calais-Germain explains in detail in *Respiration, anatomnie, geste respiratoire.*

‡ Some of these breathing techniques are nonetheless recommended for certain pathologies that affect the diaphragm or the organs around it.

REVERSE BREATHING

The belly is tucked in during inhalation and inflates during exhalation. Physiologically, this is called **"paradoxical respiration,"** which is how I will refer to it going forward. This type of breathing is nonetheless sometimes prescribed for certain pathologies (hiatal hernias, for example).

CHEST BREATHING

The belly is tucked in and permanently contracted. Certain yoga exercises encourage this sort of breathing with the specific aim of broadening expansion of the rib cage.

COLLAPSED BREATHING

High, very limited breathing, in a collapsed position. Shoulders are tucked in and the abdomen protrudes, untoned and still.

HYPERVENTILATION

Breathing that is overly fast, a possible consequence or exacerbation of chest breathing.* It can be a consequence of certain heart and kidney problems, of diabetes, or even a side effect of some medications.[18]

THROAT HOLDING

This is a similar sensation to what we feel when we are holding back a strong emotion—the urge to cry, for example. In yoga, we practice *ujjayi*, in which the glottis is closed *(see page 66).*

BREATH GRABBING

Rushing from one breath to the next without waiting to feel the need to inhale or the need to exhale.

FROZEN BREATHING

Shallow breathing, such as when we are cold and our respiratory movements are restrained by the contractions of our chest and shoulder muscles.

---

* Farhi's *The Breathing Book* notes that this might also be the result of a compensation caused by kidney disease or diabetes.

Let's Talk Through Some Essential Points

These breathing patterns all have the tendency to provoke chronic tension in the neck and shoulders, between the shoulder blades, and around the face (jaw, muscles, nose, and eyes), even causing headaches. Neither passive massage nor physical therapy will have any lasting effects on these tensions, which resume with our breathing habits.[19]

Paradoxical breathing is anti-physiological and can be difficult to identify without help. Even so, it requires rehabilitation. If you're not sure if you are breathing paradoxically, feel free to carry out the exercises in chapter 5 with a partner who can observe the movement of your breath.

Chest breathing, **collapsed breathing**, and **hyperventilation** are quite similar, but their diagnosis comes from studying the movements of the belly and rib cage. The tyranny of flat bellies and tight clothing has wreaked havoc on our bodies. In most poor breathing patterns, the belly struggles to find its proper place, curtailing the diaphragm's movement and depriving us of precious energy. Let us once again engage the full breadth of breath that our bodies were given by nature. When inhaling, we must learn—as children do and as Karlfried Graf Dürckheim[20] suggests—to "let the lower belly go." When exhaling, as Donna Farhi explains, the belly "retracts back but does not *contract*. The retraction has tone and firmness without being rigid or hard."[21]

In a permanently contracted belly, the diaphragm cannot fall. Breath dimension is limited and breathing migrates to the chest. The respiratory system's secondary muscles take over for the diaphragm and allow the ribs to expand. But this isn't their role. Even though we can't feel it—the muscles are deep inside our bodies—they tire more quickly and easily than the diaphragm.[22] Breathing becomes less efficient and the neck, shoulders, rib cage, chest, and upper back contract and grow stiff.

THE VICIOUS CIRCLE OF HYPERVENTILATION

According to some, hyperventilation is the most widespread type of dysfunctional breathing.* We generally associate it with fast, labored breathing and shortness of breath, but chronic hyperventilation is actually much subtler and can easily go unnoticed.

Hyperventilation is the degeneration of chest breathing. The breath capacity is too low and, as the body isn't getting enough oxygen, it tries to compensate by increasing our respiratory rate, the number of breaths taken per minute.

This can be the result of mouth breathing or chronic pain.[23] It can also become a habit caused by repeated exposure to stress: As the body prepares for fight or flight, our nervous system activates and gets ready to send oxygen to our muscles, therefore increasing our metabolism and dilating our blood vessels.

Under each of these circumstances, our breathing becomes faster, even though the activity we're engaged in may not require it. Having inhaled more oxygen than we need, we exhale it alongside a quantity of CO_2. And yet, our metabolism remains the same (the body is still) and, though we are exhaling fast, CO_2 production does not rise. The result is that the concentration of CO_2 in our blood plummets,[24] causing respiratory alkalosis.† The repercussions of this are complex: Our blood

---

* The physiology of hyperventilation, which author Inna Z. Khazan refers to as "overbreathing," is detailed in her book *The Clinical Handbook of Biofeedback: A Step-by-Step Guide for Training and Practice with Mindfulness.*

† Khazan notes that this phenomenon can actually occur no matter the respiratory rate and that it can be observed with the help of a capnometer, used in biofeedback to gain awareness and provide respiratory rehabilitation.

Breathe Slower, Deeper, Better

vessels contract and our oxygen supply falls; though our inhalation reflex should, in theory, be delayed, stress and lack of oxygen trigger inhalation to maintain an accelerated breathing rate. It's a vicious cycle—the more we try to breathe, the less oxygen is supplied to the body.

The physical consequences, even before they become severe, are many: vertigo, tremors, headaches, loss of focus, heart palpitations, mood swings, anxiety, and depression, not to mention the exacerbation of existing problems or illnesses. Although these symptoms have other root causes, hyperventilation is rarely thought of as one of them.

The negative effects of a permanently contracted belly can be far-reaching:

- A permanently contracted muscle becomes weak. Our muscles are designed to work in a cycle of contraction and release. So, though we may think we're making our belly stronger, we're actually doing the opposite.

- Contrary to popular belief, although strong abdominal muscles can help take the pressure off our backs, a permanently contracted abdomen will only increase tension and stiffness in the lower back. A healthy back requires a belly in motion.[25]

- The organ-stimulating massage triggered by movement of the diaphragm does not occur.

The detrimental effects of routine chest breathing, which is widespread in the West, are

- stress and/or anxiety as both cause and consequence

- accelerated and shallow breathing, as a result of limited breath capacity. This is hyperventilation. A good breathing rhythm should be
    12 to 14 breaths per minute for men
    14 to 15 breaths per minute for women
  with the ability to tolerate up to 20 breaths per minute

- heart disease or hypertension, as evidenced by numerous studies[26]

- stagnation of the lower lungs.[27]

Throat holding, breath grabbing, and **frozen breath** are narrow breathing habits. To rehabilitate them, we must draw on a deep-rooted confidence in ourselves.

Full and calm breathing is connected to finding our place on Earth.

Urging someone with poor breathing habits to "Breathe!" might result in an accentuation of the shortcomings and negative effects of their breath. The first fundamental step is to ensure that the three stages we went over in the last chapter move in sync with their breath.

Our breathing habits—if we fall into them when resting—change according to several factors, such as temperature, pain, and any substances we might ingest or inhale (stimulants, medication, poison). In the following two chapters, we will look at the influence of our bodies' position and movements—not to mention our emotions—on breathing.

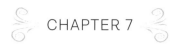

CHAPTER 7

Breathing

Position and Movement

Breathing follows movement. Though we may naturally think of movement as physical exertion, here are some other things you can try:

- Stretching *(image 12)* and contortions *(image 13)* promote breadth of inhalation.

- Lateral flexions (sideward bends) promote breadth of inhalation on the extended side and breadth of exhalation on the compacted side.

- In child's pose *(image 14)*, frontal compression of the body promotes back breathing, particularly lower-back breathing. This is also the case when lying facedown.

- When lying on your side, breathe through the top nostril.

The examples are endless. It's worth noting Jean-Pierre Laffez again: "By harmonizing breath and movement in a yoga sequence, practitioners indirectly work on their breathing."

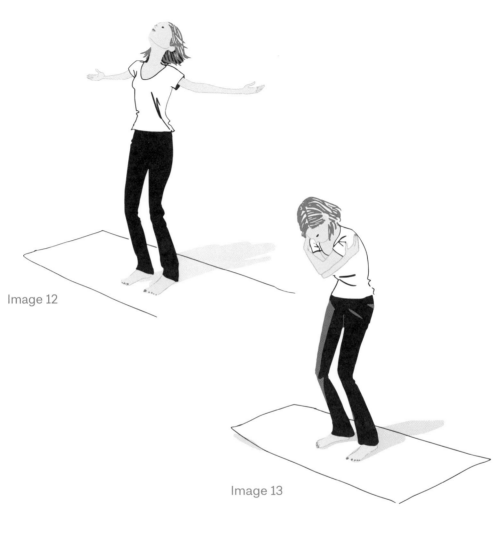

Image 12

Image 13

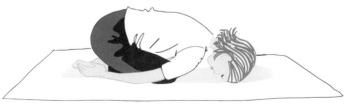

Image 14

Breathe Slower, Deeper, Better

When the movement of belly and chest is constrained by tight clothing, our breath's scope is limited. Donna Farhi warns: "If you can't run, dance, or breathe in it, don't wear it!"[28]

Let's now consider gravity's role in breathing for a body at rest.

In the lying position, the belly and chest rise on the inhalation and fall on the exhalation, as discussed in chapter 5. Once we've learned to breathe diaphragmatically in this position, what is left is to transpose this breathing method to the seated or standing position. But this transposition is not always self-evident. In the lying position, exhalation can occur in a state of full relaxation: The belly mindlessly falls under the weight of gravity. The transverse abdominal muscle, which wraps around the torso and supports the waist and lower belly, passively springs back like a rubber band under the weight of our viscera.

The measurements taken during the first two parts of Test 1 are reasonable indications of your automatic breathing habits and should allow you, in principle, to reach the following conclusion:

- During inhalation, movement around the waist is noticeably the same when lying down as it is when sitting up. This can be explained by the fact that the impact of the diaphragm's movement on the areas surrounding it is greater than that of gravity. In the resting position, the effect of an inhalation on the pelvic floor is gentle—it does not require it to contract.

- Around the waist, in the lying position, is where the breadth of movement from inhalation to exhalation is at its greatest. These variations in inhalation and exhalation are weakest around the lower waist.

- The measurements taken between the lying and seated position—around the lower waist—illustrate the effects of gravity, confirming the importance of a toned abdomen and of the transverse abdominals' contraction during exhalation, when seated or standing.

- The disparity in the measurements taken around the lower waist during inhalation and exhalation in the seated position will give you an idea of your transverse abdominal muscle's elasticity and firmness. If there is no disparity, your belly is either permanently tensed or slack.

Now that you've learned to loosen your belly to breathe better in the lying position, you should avoid falling into sloppy habits while standing, which could lead you to succumb to the type of collapsed breathing covered in chapter 6, in which the belly remains slack and untoned. This is often evident in overly sedentary, obese, or depressed people, though it can happen to anyone. The belly bulges during inhalation and remains passive during exhalation. The abs do not fulfill their role, so gravity pulls the bulging belly down, softens the abdominal muscles, and slumps the posture while tugging at the lumbar spine. This interferes with the diaphragm's rise, which makes exhalation less efficient and restricts breathing. This worsens with age and with the loss of the muscle elasticity and tone. Not very sexy, right?

With the torso in a vertical position, we will need to confirm or, if need be, introduce **an essential element: the transverse abdominal muscle's exertion during exhalation.**[*] Why this abdominal muscle in particular?

---

[*] Bernadette de Gasquet, in *Abs: Stop the Massacre!*, expresses this as follows: "The more the abdominal wall is slack, the greater the risk of the abdominal muscles flopping forwards. With the spine at the back supporting upright posture, the viscera automatically tend to move forwards and downwards due to the forces of gravity."

Because it's the only muscle that, instead of forcing the torso to bend when it contracts, helps our posture remain erect. As such, the belly, retracting during exhalation—without reaching maximal expiration—can follow the diaphragm as it rises again, just like in the lying position. This is what had been missing from my breathing all this time, and it took me a long time to understand it.

There are several ways to create a spontaneous breathing habit in which the toned transverse abdominal muscle contracts during exhalation.

- Contract the transverse abdominal muscle and lift the pelvic floor. You can associate it with certain activities throughout the day, so that you think about it regularly (waiting for red lights or when standing in line, for example).

- Remember to relax the pelvic floor gently.

- Strengthen your abs through basic abdominal exercises.

- In chapter 9, I suggest a few yoga exercises in which a deep exhalation automatically works the transverse abdominal muscle.*

Our goal is to find a midpoint between a permanently tight, hard, and rigid belly and one that is slack, flabby, and soft. In other words, we want a toned belly that moves with our breath. "With it," according to the late, great yoga instructor Loredana Hamoniaux, "your breathing sensations will not fall but instead prosper effortlessly and radiate throughout the entire body."[29]

We've now looked at the effects of movement and position on breathing. But the opposite is also true: **Breathing influences position.**

---

* For those familiar with the form of "madras" breathing taught by T. K. V. Desikachar and Yoga de l'Énergie's *movement de liaison* will have positive effects on your abdominal muscles, especially the transverse muscle.

We don't often do this in the day-to-day, but it is possible to breathe voluntarily with a specific part of the lungs. For example, by intentionally inhaling through your left side and exhaling through your right, your spine will gradually lean rightward. It might be helpful to place your hands on your ribs when doing so (images 15a and 15b). It may take several breaths before you can feel your body tilt. Do the same on the other side to balance it out.*

If you intentionally inhale through the front of the body, your torso will naturally straighten and correct a hunched posture. This is a key ingredient in the search for our standing body's proper positioning.

Do certain positions or particular situations require less oxygen? Yes, sleep and meditation do because our bodies and minds are both at rest. Our breathing, as always, adapts to circumstance. When the brain is active—during REM sleep or when the mind has once again taken over after meditation—our oxygen needs increase, again changing how we breathe.

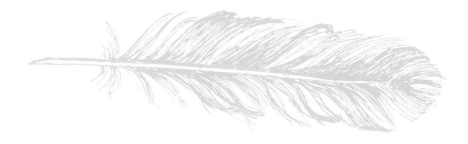

---

* I owe this exercise and the discovery of this bodily skill to Patrick Tomatis, a renowned yoga instructor.

Breathe Slower, Deeper, Better

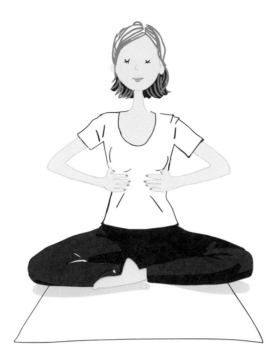

Image 15a

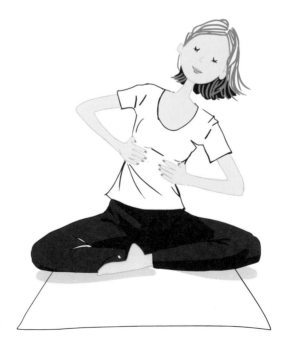

Image 15b

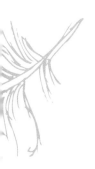

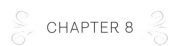

CHAPTER 8

Breathing and Emotions

Though yogic texts speak more of the mind than emotions, the two are closely related. Emotions, which are housed in the body, are mental emanations.

Taittiriya Upanishad, an Indian text that dates to approximately 600 BCE, describes man as a series of bodies or concentric sheaths or layers (the *koshas*). This is one of the foundations of yoga philosophy. The sheaths are, from the coarsest to the subtlest, the outermost to the most intimate.

- *Annamaya kosha:* food

- *Pranamaya kosha:* vital breath

- *Manomaya kosha:* mind

- *Vijñānmāyā kosha:* discernment or intellect

- *Anandamaya kosha:* heart, love, and light

Two consecutive sheaths interact, creating numerous connections. Let's explore the connection between the second and third sheaths: the breath and the mind.

A later text, *The Hatha Yoga Pradipika,* makes this connection explicit: "When the breath is unsteady, the mind is unsteady . . ." (II, 2). And later, "He who binds the breath, binds the mind. He who binds the mind, binds the breath" (IV, 21). More than mere interaction, these statements imply the possibility of a voluntary and conscious action by the breath on the mind. This is fairly well-recognized today. The text goes even further, laying out a structured technique that can be used to master the breath: the pranayama.

BREATHING IS IMMEDIATELY ALTERED AS SOON AS THERE IS A CHANGE WITHIN US OR IN THE WORLD AROUND US, SEEMING ALMOST TO ANTICIPATE EACH CHANGE.

—JEAN-PIERRE LAFFEZ[30]

Our inner state and emotions, which stem from the mind, are reflected in how we breathe and have a multitude of other effects on our bodies: change in heart rate, perspiration, tremor, excitement, throat tightening, stomach cramps, blushing. In contrast, our breath is the only thing we can directly affect.

There is a type of breathing for each emotion. "We don't breathe the same when we are happy, in pain, with a friend, an enemy, or even with someone we love."[31] What's more, there's a command center for each respiratory action: normal breathing, yawning, coughing, sighing.[32]

The main correlations between emotions, sensations, and breathing types are as follows:

- Joy, associated with laughter, is a succession of short, noisy exhalations.

Breathe Slower, Deeper, Better

- Sadness, associated with crying, is a succession of small inhalations.

- Fear, like cold, causes frozen breath or even apnea.

- Anger incites a noisy breath, often a deep inhalation preceding an eruption (loud voice, yelling).

The day I realized that I'd been trying to contain my anger with deep inhalations and that the effect of this was exactly the opposite of what I'd intended, I took a big step* to change my behavior. I replaced that deep inhalation with a protracted exhalation that allowed me to calm down enough to express myself without yelling.

- Surprise is a pause in breath or a noisy aspiration through the mouth, depending on the intensity of emotion.

- Relief and frustration are associated with sighing. But there are different kinds of sighs. While a frustrated sigh is a willful, noisy exhalation, a sigh of relief is an inhalation that extends into a deeper inhalation, followed by an exhalation where "the lungs' elasticity returns unrestrained. The sigh is therefore both a witness to and a means by which to relax the body, in particular the diaphragm. It promotes rest, relaxation, fluidity."[33]

- Well-being, relaxation, and surrender are associated with yawning, which is a deep inhalation followed by a muscle spasm that pulls down the lower jaw. A yawn can be a sign of fatigue. It is said to balance pressure as well as oxygen intake and to provoke the secretion of an endorphin which places the body at rest.

* When my three children were young, they were active and quarreled often. Yoga had already helped me figure out that the reason I reacted that way was more than just my kids' behavior. Whenever I went to yoga in the mornings, our afternoons were much better!

- Another sensation, the great struggle of our times: stress, an age-old reflex to danger. Though we still need it today, it grips us more often than is necessary. Originally meant as a reaction to a threat that would induce a fight-or-flight response, in our modern lives it has become an accumulation of reactions to a variety of stimuli. Stress can be stimulating or inhibiting, depending on whether we actively respond to the situation. The type of breathing associated with stress is often high, fast, and narrow.

Through breath, we can calm our minds and soothe our emotions. It's a tool at once childishly simple—all you have to do is breathe!—and extraordinarily complicated. We all know how difficult it can be to master our emotions with our minds.

Breathing is such a powerful mechanism that it can even generate emotions. Actors simulate an emotion by engaging with the corresponding breath. For example, to incite joy or laughter, they resort to a series of exhalations, which is something laughter yoga also proposes. A calming breath then helps to take a step back from these provoked emotions. A calming breath can also help to manage stage fright.

But a calming breath, which can affect any emotion and soothes stress, isn't just any breath. For a breath to be calming, it has to be full but also forceful, regular, and fluid, with a long exhalation that doesn't leave you breathless. This appeals to the parasympathetic nervous system, which calms the body by keeping it at its base metabolism, at its most sedate.[*]

A protracted exhalation is crucial. Roger Clerc,[†] in his teaching, often raised the need to "completely empty before refilling." Practice this by

---

[*] Notes taken during Andrée Maman's breathing course at EFY. Andrée Maman is a radiologist who followed the teachings of T. K. V. Desikachar, a great Indian yoga instructor.

[†] A great instructor who disseminated the teachings of Yoga de l'Energie in France.

exhaling deeply, blowing out through a partly open mouth, then consciously awaiting the need to inhale.

A few calming breaths can be enough to change the way we view a situation. By placing a hand on your belly, you can speed up the soothing process.

EXAM STRESS

I often share this breathing technique, from Mr. Mény, my math teacher, which helped me during my studies.

- One two-count* inhalation

- One two-count pause

- One three-count exhalation

When breathing is simultaneously delicate, focused, conscious, and located in the physical and energetic body, it can reach beyond—to a place of subtlety, presence, and openness, of acceptance and looseness, until, finally, we renounce all the expectations we might have felt around it.

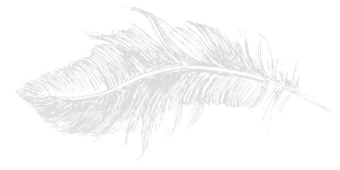

* We'll later return to this "count," which lasts about one second, but can be adapted by each individual to ensure a comfortable practice for the duration of each respiratory phase.

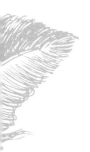

CHAPTER 9

Breathing Exercises

As soon as we start observing our breath, it becomes conscious and changes.

The overall impact of yogic breathing exercises is as follows: improved diaphragm mobility, lung capacity, and blood circulation—and, therefore, improved oxygenation of the entire body. The following exercises will lighten the work done by your heart and promote good health by appealing to the parasympathetic nervous system. By soothing the mind, you can reduce negative emotions—stress, anxiety, depression, anger, fear—as well as compulsive or addictive behaviors.

The exercises in this chapter, most of which stem from yoga tradition, are relatively straightforward. Their goal is to make the three stages move in sync with our breath, lengthening each phase, particularly exhalation, and introducing breath suspensions. Each exercise comes with step-by-step instructions, possible variations, and a note on adverse effects, as well as specific outcomes.

These exercises can be practiced in sequence (this will take about half an hour) or individually, depending on the time you have at your disposal.

In the case of the latter, you should try to respect the suggested order. These exercises can be seen as preparation for pranayama, which systematically incorporates suspensions of breath, as well as mudras (position of hands or tongue) and *bandhas* ("body locks" that allow you to keep energy in your torso). It might be interesting to integrate them incrementally into a meditative practice that does not include breathwork.

A fundamental, physiological rule of pranayama is that **the duration of an exhalation should always be longer or equal to that of the inhalation.**[*] Generally speaking, yoga promotes exhalation and breath suspensions: Aphorism I, 34, from *The Yoga-Sutra of Patañjali* effectively says that "the mind may be calmed by expulsion and retention of the breath." Try to follow this rule in the exercises to come.

By using variations of these four counts of breathing, you can create breathing rhythms[†] that are

- **Toned and stimulating:** The full-lung suspension should be longer than the empty-lung suspension.

    Inhalation + full-lung suspension > exhalation + empty-lung suspension
    Example: The 2:2:3:0 rhythm in the box on page 53 (the durations correspond to the differences in the four breathing phases).

- **Calming and soothing:** Exhalation should be longer than inhalation.

    Inhalation + full-lung suspension < exhalation + empty-lung suspension
    Example: 3:2:5:2 rhythm, which is used a lot in Yoga de l'Énergie.

[*†] Notes taken in Andrée Maman's course on breathing at EFY.

- **Balanced:** Duration of inhalation and exhalation should be identical, as are suspensions.

  Inhalation + full-lung suspension = exhalation + empty-lung suspension
  Example: A 2:1:2:1 rhythm, a good base starting rhythm, which
  shows that both sides are equal.

The effects of these exercises last for some time, and with repetition, we can establish a balanced new breathing habit and help it take root more permanently. By gaining awareness throughout the day of how we breathe (or taking a break for a few deep breaths), we can relearn how to breathe and start to adopt better habits.

This new breathing method will take us to another level: As we inhale and exhale air, a subtle energy—prana—courses through us. It's only when we're connected to this reality that we are truly breathing. "Breath evokes the manifestation of a power that pierces the flesh and mind and is then translated into energy. All the while, it remains impossible or illicit to appropriate it. Man doesn't make breath, he receives it."[34] We can therefore bear witness to the fact that "it breathes in us." This prana is the equivalent of the One, the Absolute, and of Pure Consciousness.*

Advice Before You Begin

- Wait two to three hours after eating.

- Set aside a quiet time for yourself in which you won't be interrupted. Find a room large enough for you to lay down a rug or mat. Get ahold of the necessary material for each exercise.

---

* According to *Kaushitaki Upanishad*, "Prana is Brahman" (II, 1 and 2), "Life is prana, prana is life . . . As long as prana dwells in the body, so long surely there is life" (III, 3).

- Begin by preparing your body with yoga that moves your spine and abdominals in every direction. As discussed, a strong abdominal wall is a precious breathing ally. In Patañjali's Royal Yoga, pranayama goes hand in hand with postural practice (and precedes meditation).

- Respect your own rhythm, focus on the exactness of what you're practicing while also listening to your body, your best guide. You'll sense when to adapt the exercises to your needs. This practice should not make you tired during or after. Don't force it; don't compete against yourself. Instead seek flexibility and gentleness, which is just as important as, if not more than, postural practice. When executed poorly, pranayama can lead to gastrointestinal problems, hypertension, and even nervous breakdowns.[35] *The Hatha Yoga Pradipika* (II, 16) is even more categorical, "Correct pranayama will weaken all diseases. Improper practice of Yoga will strengthen all diseases."

- Work gradually so that you become familiar with your new breath. Opt for exhalation and yawning, which go hand in hand with surrender, letting go, making space, and respecting our bodies.

- Don't hesitate to ask a qualified yoga instructor for advice. They can answer your questions, detect possible adverse effects, and adjust your practice. It's not unusual to see people who think they're properly positioned and moving correctly, both in terms of posture and breath, who are actually unaware of their mistakes.

- Seek medical advice for specific illnesses (such as asthma, hypertension, epilepsy, hyperventilation syndrome, and all other disorders relating to the respiratory system or are located near the diaphragm, such as hiatal hernias).

- If practicing at a studio where the duration of each breathing phase is determined by the instructor's voice or a metronome and is too long for you, don't hesitate to adapt accordingly.

Child's Pose

Child's pose (a translation of the Sanskrit term *balasana*)
is also called "folded leaf." I recommend beginning with this
pose because it promotes internal centering and will make the
lying position in the following exercises more comfortable,
thanks to the lower back stretch.

SETTLING INTO THE POSITION

Sit on your heels. While exhaling, fold your spine and head forward. Stretch your arms back and rest them on the ground with your elbows and the backs of your hands on the floor *(image 16)*. Your entire body should be relaxed (be sure to relax your face, too). This position requires no physical exertion.

This should be a comfortable position. If it isn't, try the following variation.

Variation *(image 17):* Extend your arms in front of you. This is a firmer position because your shoulders are stretched and your arm muscles are engaged in an isometric contraction.

EXERCISE

Observe the point where your belly and thighs connect. You might feel a slight pressure due to the belly's compression. By shifting your attention to your back, you will discover pleasant, open, and free back breathing that requires no movement. This is a way of experiencing that great natural law— in which one thing closes, and something else opens—in our bodies. The point is to figure out exactly where this is happening.

DURATION

Focus on back breathing for a few minutes.

VARIATIONS

- If your ankles hurt or feel stiff, place a rolled-up towel beneath them.

- If your knees hurt, place a thin blanket or cushion between your buttocks and calves.

- If the pressure is too uncomfortable, spread your knees, widening the distance between them.

- If your head doesn't reach the floor and you feel unsettled, place your head on a cushion or on your wrists, with one stacked above the other.

- If you are pregnant, adapt this position by spreading your knees and extending your arms forward.

POSITIVE EFFECTS

Revitalizes and soothes the mind. Thanks to gravity, this posture works hip and knee flexibility and stretches your forefoot. It soothes the cervical spine and stimulates circulation of blood to your head. The fold also stretches your back.

ADVERSE EFFECTS

Knee pain.

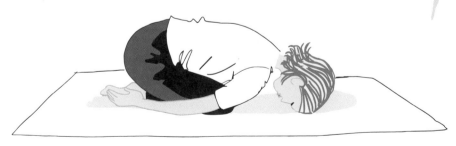

Image 16

Breathe Slower, Deeper, Better

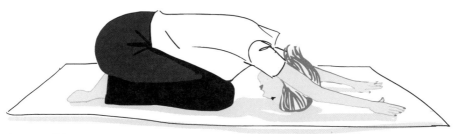

Image 17

The Three Stages of Breathing

Now that you're familiar with this exercise, feel free to shorten it:
After settling comfortably into this position and relaxing,
rest your arms by your side as you grow aware of the three
breathing stages, as discussed in chapter 5. Then, take
three breaths with help from your arms.

POSITIVE EFFECTS

Rehabilitation of the movement of the three stages of breathing. Broadening of breathing movements and increased lung capacity, which has multiple benefits: improved tissue oxygenation, healing, stress abatement, improved resistance to negative emotions. Prana leads to an openness toward life and a joie de vivre.

Exhalation Work with Pelvic Floor

An excellent exercise proposed by Blandine Calais-Germain[36]
for all ages, starting at puberty.

POSITION

Lie on your back with knees bent and feet parallel to each other, planted on
the floor near your pelvis. Your feet and knees should be hip-width apart,
arms a short distance from body with palms facing upward *(image 18)*.

ADJUSTMENT

If your back is arched and your lower back is not touching the floor, press
your feet down harder on the floor when exhaling. You should feel a pleasant
sensation as your lower back touches the floor.

EXERCISE

Following a deep inhalation, exhale upward from your pelvic floor. Contract
the pelvic floor (a rising sensation), then clench your belly from bottom to top
(engaging your transverse abdominal muscle) until the end of your exhalation.
The pelvic floor should gently relax before and during the inhalation.

Each of the following four sounds must be repeated three times, each
followed by one or two deep breaths to ensure the pelvic floor is relaxed. If
you're new to this, it might help to know that you should register a different
sensation between the end of an exhalation and the inhalation.

At every stage, exhalation is accompanied by a sound:

- A whistling "s" sound

- A whistling "f" sound

- An "ah" sound, as if blowing on a glass, mouth wide open

- Coughing. In this last stage, you will feel your pelvic floor and belly contract simultaneously, which is entirely normal due to the rapid exhalation. This cough-exhalation protects the pelvic floor. Until it becomes automatic, try to think of contracting the pelvic floor whenever you feel you're going to cough, laugh, or sneeze *(see chapter 4)*.

Rest for a few moments so that you can enjoy the effects of the exercise, then take deep breaths with the help of your arms *(see page 33)*. Yawning or tearing up is a good sign.

To leave this position, bring one knee then the other up to your belly, then roll onto your side to sit up.

POSITIVE EFFECTS

Works deep muscles in contraction-release cycle, which tones the pelvic floor, preventing bladder weakness, prolapse in women, and prostate and erectile dysfunction in men. It also helps to maintain a healthy sexual life. By coordinating pelvic floor movements with your breathing, this exercise activates and exercises your focus and concentration, fostering a deep and meaningful relaxation.

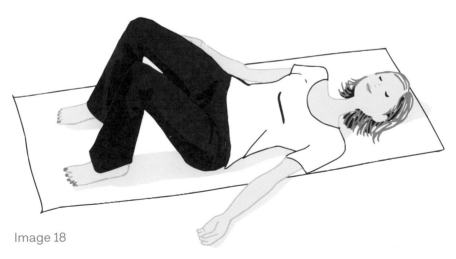

Image 18

SETTLING INTO A SEATED POSITION

Find a comfortable seated position by placing a pillow on the floor, and sit on your knees with a pillow between your thighs and calves, or sit on a small stool or chair. If this isn't comfortable enough, set up some pillows against the wall or the back of your chair, and keep your back upright.

The pelvis will be slightly tilted forward and your weight distributed equally. Legs should be comfortably relaxed, your back straight, and the shoulders relaxed, low, and open.

Become aware of your vertical axis, which extends from your perineum to the tip of your cranium. Breathe a few times between these two points, rising with your inhalation and lowering with your exhalation so that you can better visualize and feel it.

Move your attention to the opening of your nostrils, keeping your breathing natural.

A posture that is initially comfortable risks becoming the opposite. Although the following exercises all take place in a seated position, don't hesitate to modify it if you feel uncomfortable.

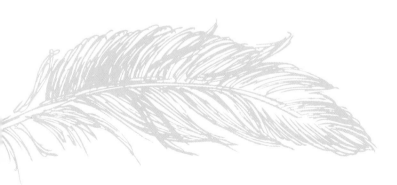

Breathe Slower, Deeper, Better

Pranic Breathing

This breathing method is slow and conscious. It involves a very delicate inhalation—as if sniffing perfume—and engages our sense of smell. With this breath, says Roger Clerc, "we become aware of the fact that the air we breathe holds not only oxygen, which is indispensable to life . . . but an energy that sends vibrations through the primordial material that we and life are made of."[37]

EXERCISE

Inhale, and follow your breath's path from the tip of your nose to its root, between both eyebrows, and then exhale, feeling the air leaving your nostrils, both inside and outside, as well as along your upper lip. Then stop, and tune into the faint sound of your breath as the air enters and leaves. Your sense of smell, touch, and hearing are alert.

DURATION

Ten or so breaths, or until these subtle sensations have taken root.

POSITIVE EFFECTS

Eminently calming. It slows the breath, increases awareness of our relationship with the air, the environment, and the world around us.

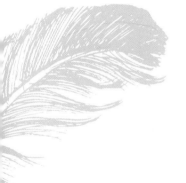

Ujjayi Breathing

The "victorious breath" should be practiced with a closed mouth during both inhalation and exhalation, with the glottis remaining tight. Airflow is restricted and the breath lengthens.

EXERCISE

Preparation: With your mouth open, breathe as though you are exhaling onto a chilled piece of glass, as if to create condensation (as we did above by emitting an "ah" from the throat). As you do this, try to constrict your windpipe to achieve a clearly perceptible sound.

Try to reproduce these sensations, now with your mouth closed during both inhalation and exhalation. Though fainter, the sound should still be present. Resembling waves, it's sometimes referred to as "ocean breath."

DURATION

Ten or so breaths.

POSITIVE EFFECTS

A protracted exhalation sets the mind at ease. This breathing is excellent preparation for public speaking because it both cleans the vocal cords and reduces stress, promoting a sure, well-placed voice. It can help soothe tonsillitis and recurring hiccups, as well as reduce snoring, chronic chills, and asthma.[38] The *Gheranda Samhita* also notes that this type of breathing has positive effects on nervous disorders, indigestion, cold, and fevers.

ADVERSE EFFECTS

Irritated throat, infection of the nasopharynx.

A Balancing Breath

This breath can be used for energy and wellness.
Channel it to the parts of your body that are stiff or
painful. You'll see how powerful an intention can be.

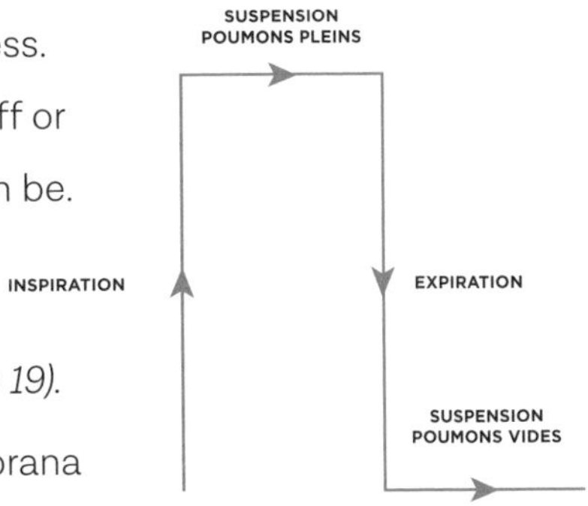

EXERCISE

The recommended rhythm here is 2:1:2:1 *(image 19)*.

- Inhalation (two-count): Become aware of prana
  as it enters and fills your entire body.

- Full-lung suspension (one-count): Centered in the
  torso, prana takes the shape of energy and wellness.

- Exhalation (two-count): Prana disperses throughout the body.

- Full-lung suspension (one-count): Full relaxation and surrender.

SUSPENSION
POUMONS PLEINS

INSPIRATION

EXPIRATION

SUSPENSION
POUMONS VIDES

Image 19

DURATION

Ten breaths.

POSITIVE EFFECTS

Balancing, due to its rhythm. For the exercises with longer inhalations than
exhalations, this breathing allows the breath to softly lengthen while toning the
abdominal muscles. By increasing concentration of CO_2, the full-lung suspension
can benefit those who suffer from chronic hyperventilation *(see page 38)*.

ADVERSE EFFECTS

Avoid breath suspensions in cases of heart problems, or if they make you
feel unwell or suffocated. Avoid doing this exercise before bedtime if your
exhalations are naturally longer than your inhalations, either spontaneously or
due to your practice, as this may be invigorating and cause sleeping problems.

Kapalabhati

The breath that "makes the skull shine" is one of the six purification exercises that are the foundation of traditional hatha yoga (the *shat kriyas*). This exercise precedes pranayama. Inhalation and exhalation alternate quickly "like the bellows of a blacksmith," per *The Hatha Yoga Pradipika* (II, 35). This breathing method emphasizes exhalation, which grows active while inhalation becomes passive *(images 20a and 20b)*. Exhalations are strong, like sneezing several times in a row or trying to blow out a candle with your nose.

PREPARATION

If you're unfamiliar with this exercise, place a hand on your belly to check that it is moving correctly. It is imperative for your belly to retract during the rapid exhalation, so make sure you are not breathing paradoxically.

In the beginning, take time to inhale fully before exhaling again, then step up the rhythm little by little. If you breathe too quickly to settle into a rapid rhythm, you risk rushing your inhalation and not really letting the belly relax between exhalations. It is worth training with a yoga instructor before making this part of your regular practice.

EXERCISE

The pelvic floor should remain toned (mildly tensed) for the duration of this exercise. Consider releasing it afterward.

Take twenty breaths. Start slowly, letting this movement take root: Inhale deeply after each rapid exhalation.

Once you've become familiar with this movement, you'll do three twenty-breath sequences, with one deep breath in between. Once you're done, take some time to absorb these sensations and observe the effects of your breath within you. After taking your final breath, pay particular attention to the natural extension of your exhalation and empty-lung suspension.

LET YOUR ATTENTION REST DEEPLY ON THE PAUSE
AT THE END OF THE OUTGOING BREATH. THIS IS THE ORIGIN
OF THE BREATH, WHERE THE BREATH ARISES AND WHERE
THE BREATH RETURNS TO. LET YOUR ENTIRE BEING FALL
BACK INTO THE PAUSE, TRUSTING THAT THE NEW BREATH
WILL ARISE WITHOUT ANY EFFORT ON YOUR PART.[39]
—DONNA FARHI

POSITIVE EFFECTS

Cleansing, intense abdominal workout. This is one of the most effective exercises for recovering the natural contraction of your abdominal transverse muscle, and therefore belly retraction during exhalation. It warms the respiratory system and facilitates empty-lung breath suspension. After practicing, the breath becomes naturally longer, and the mind stabilizes.

ADVERSE EFFECTS

Paradoxical breathing; pelvic-floor weakness for pregnant, postpartum, and menstruating women; heart problems; hypertension; hypotension; emotional sensitivity; hyperventilation syndrome.

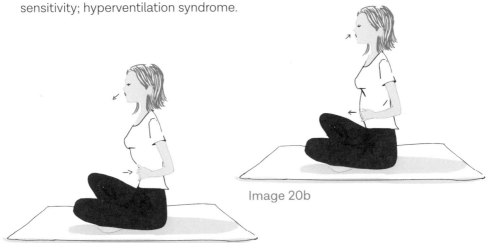

Image 20b

Image 20a

Alternate Nostril Breathing

Preparation for *nadī̇́ shodhana pranayama,*
"channel-cleaning breath."

HAND POSITION

Use your right thumb and ring finger to alternately close your nostrils: Place your thumb on your right nostril and your ring finger on your left nostril. Your pinkie finger should meet your ring finger effortlessly. Traditionally, there are two designated positions for the index and middle fingers, which remain together:

- They can rest on the forehead; this is easiest for beginners *(image 21a).*

- They can fold into the fleshy part of the thumb in *nasika mudra (image 21b),* with the palm of the hand being partly closed.

The left hand, which you can use to set up the right hand, rests on the knee in *chin mudra* (tips of thumb and index finger touch, with the remaining fingers held together).

EXERCISE

The following sequence, which starts after an inhalation through both nostrils, is how I was first taught:

- Left exhalation (right nostril closed)

- Left inhalation (right nostril closed)

- Right exhalation (left nostril closed)

- Right inhalation (left nostril closed)

Start this cycle over or end with an exhalation through both nostrils.

OBSERVATIONS

The beginning and end of this breathing technique vary from one line of yoga to the next. If physically able, you may sit in lotus, or *padmasana,* as prescribed by *The Hatha Yoga Pradipika* (see top of next page). But, thankfully, sitting in lotus isn't a prerequisite for breathing correctly.

ADVANCE IN STAGES

1. Start with ten breaths and no breath suspensions (five cycles).
2. Once you've established a regular breathing rhythm that is gentle and full, try to lengthen your exhalation. It might help to count, but only once your breath is regular, to keep from constraining it.
3. Implement a full-lung suspension (the only one in this pranayama) by starting with one count then gradually increasing, without force.

POSITIVE EFFECTS

Balances out airflow between nostrils, strengthens immune system, alternately stimulates both hemispheres of the brain, and soothes the mind. Closing off one nostril helps lengthen the breath. The energetic effect of this pranayama is, as its name indicates, to cleanse and balance the two nadis, *ida* and *pingala*. It balances the opposing pairs within us (such as hot and cold, material and spiritual, sympathetic and parasympathetic nervous systems).

VARIATION

If you can't breathe through one nostril, set both hands on your knees. You can practice through visualization, through pure and simple concentration.

THE YOGI, HAVING ASSUMED PADMASANA, SHOULD INHALE PRANA WITH THE MOON. AFTER HOLDING AS LONG AS POSSIBLE, HE SHOULD EXHALE WITH THE SUN. HE SHOULD FILL THE INTERIOR SLOWLY BY INHALING PRANA WITH THE SUN. AFTER HOLDING IN THE PRESCRIBED MANNER, HE SHOULD EXHALE WITH THE MOON.*

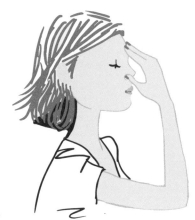

Image 21a

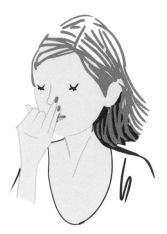

Image 21b

---

* *The Hatha Yoga Pradipika*, II, 7–8. Here, "moon" and "sun" refer respectively to the left, feminine side (*tha* in hatha yoga) and to the right, masculine side (*ha* in hatha yoga).

Breathe Slower, Deeper, Better

Om

This is yoga's simplest mantra, the most used and powerful, though its symbolism is unknown. In Sanskrit, *o* is the contraction of *a* and *u* ("oo") and can be sung as "aum" or "om."

MANTRA

Sing three *a*'s, three *u*'s ("oo"), and three *m*'s (closed mouth), followed by three *aum*'s. Dwell on the sensations these vibrations create by shifting your attention to where they are most evident: the top of the skull, the mouth, the whole head, and then the entire body.

OBSERVATIONS

Every person must find their own note, which can vary depending on the day, moment, or mood. Sometimes, you have to search for the right frequency. In a group, you're under no obligation to sing like the person next to you; any feelings of dissonance should be overcome so that the note feels just right to each person, without being forced.

POSITIVE EFFECTS

Lengthens breath. Automatically works abdominal muscles, as in singing. "When feeling frustrated," Guy Taïeb says, "our vibration frequency is disturbed. Singing om moves our entire being back toward the proper vibration frequency, like tuning an instrument." Singing om solidifies our sense of being, vibrant and boundless, larger than we are.

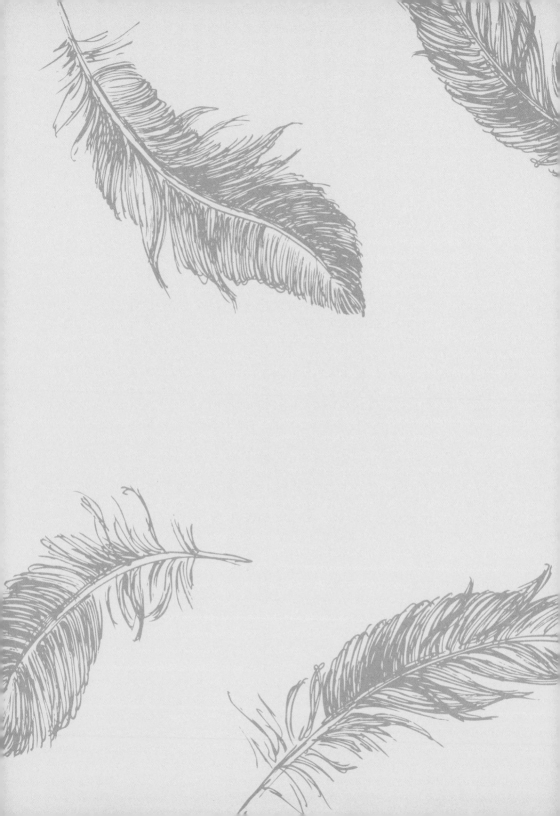

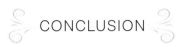

Breathing, a gesture we have engaged in continuously since birth, impacts our health, well-being, and energy, as well as our minds and emotions. We have developed a breathing pattern all our own, which resurfaces automatically when we breathe unconsciously. This breathing pattern may be spontaneous, but there's nothing natural about it. It can be observed, studied at will, rehabilitated. Yoga philosophy is optimistic: Every person has the ability to replace their bad habits with healthier ones, even though doing so isn't often quick or easy.

With a little awareness, training, and perseverance, we can breathe and live better: Physically, with better overall wellness—you should be able to feel a change as early as your first practice—emotionally, with an easy mind that is more resistant to stress, and spiritually, with a new way of being in the world.

By developing well-placed, calm, broad, supple, slow, and harmonious breathing, we can access a new away of living that is subtler and more vibrant, that can be felt along the entire surface of our skin, throughout our whole body. Breathing becomes breath. Prana courses through us, a breath that opens up and wraps us in confidence and joy instead of shuttering and isolating us in fear.

It is quite normal for you to find that you are "obsessed" with your breathing after reading this book. But if you have glimpsed the truth of Roger Clerc's description of breathing as "the art of vibrating in harmony with everything," you'll have discovered something truly special.

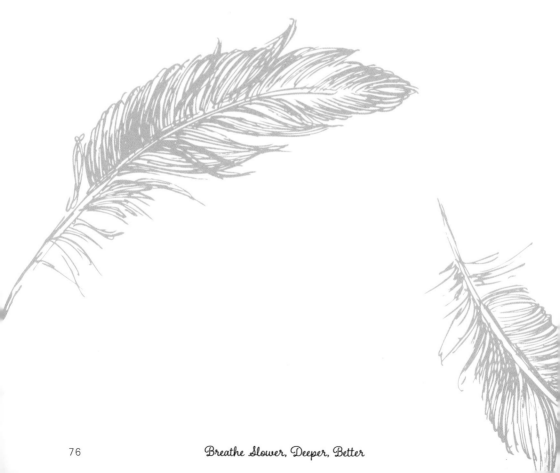

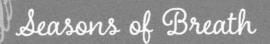

Seasons of Breath

I am dawn rising, Life murmuring,
Fluttering, vulnerable and potent,
The dew on the flower, the echo of the first howl,
A sprout bent on breaking through the tar.

I am day and light cast on action deployed,
Mountain reaching to heaven,
A choice amid possibility, a drive for legacy,
The brisk feeling of scattered time.

I am the final breath, engulfed cliff,
Supreme repose, the smoothness of waves,
The surrender of all that is material and gained.
The world contracting in contemplation.

I am the long night slumbering in silence,
A buried seed, the soul in suspense.
A return to the Source, alert, latent, patient,
You who wager over me, I am that which watches over.

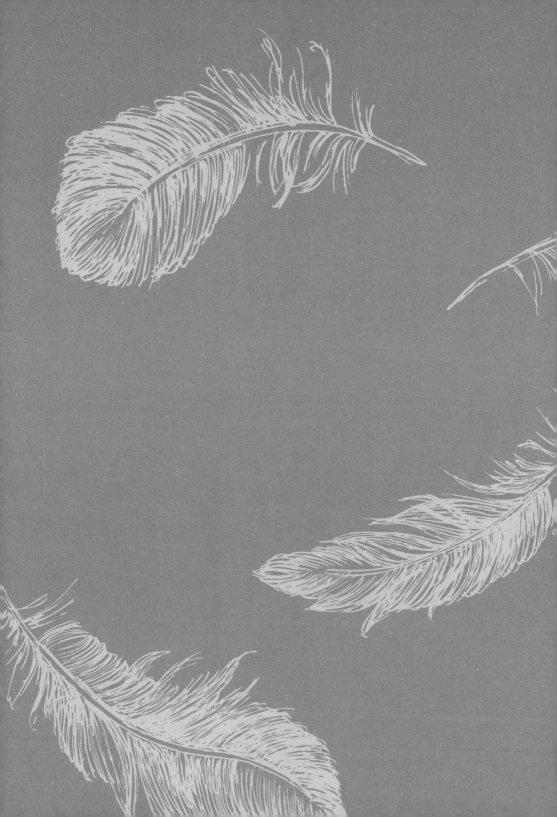

ENDNOTES

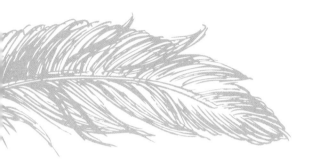

1. Calais-German, Blandine. *Respiration, anatomie, geste respiratoire*. Gap, France: Désiris, 2005 (73).

2. Durand, Maud. Interview with Jean-Pierre Laffez. "L'art de respirer est une clé pour notre santé." *La Vie*, no. 3742 (May 2017): 23.

3. Taïeb, Guy. Notes from the conference "De la respiration" (On Breathing), November 19, 2016, in Fontenay-le-Fleury, France.

4. Ibid.

5. *The Yoga Sutras of Patañjali*. Translated by Edwin F. Bryant. New York: North Point Press, 2009.

6. Farhi, Donna. *The Breathing Book: Good Health and Vitality Through Essential Breath Work*. New York: St. Martin's Griffin, 1996 (51).

7. Ibid., 53.

8. Durand and Laffez, "L'art de respire est une clé pour notre santé," 22.

9. Laffez, Jean-Pierre. *La Respiration, notions de physiologie appliquée*, EFY handouts (59).

10. Farhi, *The Breathing Book*, 53.

11. Laffez, *La Respiration, notions de physiologie appliquée*, 33.

12. Gaucet, Béatrice. "La respiration dans le chant classique," *La Voie du souffle*, Revue Française de Yoga, no. 28, 2003: 139.

13. Clerc, Roger. *La Respiration, contrôle du souffle, manières et art de respire, l'art de vibrer à l'unison du tout*. Paris, France: Le Courrier de Livre, 1995 (13).

14. Jeze, Françoise. "L'utilisation du souffle dans un processes analytique," *La Voie du souffle*. Revue Française de Yoga, no. 28 (August 2003): 155. Published by FNEY (Fédération Nationale des Enseignants de Yoga).

15. Arnold Gesell, as quoted by Jean-Pierre Laffez in "Biomécanique de la respiration," *La Voie du souffle*, 102.

16. Leccia, Marie-Christine. "Étude du pranayama à travers quelquers textes traditionnels indiens," *La Voie du souffle*, 26.

17. Farhi, *The Breathing Book*, 74–92.

18. Khazan, Inna Z. *The Clinical Handbook of Biofeedback: A Step-by-Step Guide for Training and Practice with Mindfulness*. Malden, MA: John Wiley & Sons, 2013 (77).

19. Ibid., 58.

20. Karlfried Graf Dürckheim, *Le Centre de l'être*, Albin Michel, 155.

21. Farhi, *The Breathing Book*, 25.

22. Ibid., 49, 58.

23. Ibid., 76.

24. Ibid., 78.

25. Ibid., 40.

26. Ibid., 59.

27. Ibid., 116.

28. Ibid., 96.

29. Hamoniaux, Loredana. "Asana, méditation musculaire," *Les carnets du yoga*, no. 353 (January 2017).

30. Laffez, *La Respiration, notions de physiologie appliquée*, 94.

31. Ibid., 92.

32. Demorand, Stéphane. "Soupirez, c'est bon pour la santé!," lepoint.fr (November 27, 2017).

33. Calais-Germain, *Respiration, anatomie, geste respiratoire*, 152.

34. Tardan-Masquelier, Ysé. "Le souffle et la vie spirituelle dans les grands traditions d'Orient." *La Voie du souffle*, 160.

35. *Pranayama: The Science of Breathing in Mind Management*, 4th ed. Chennai: Vivekananda Kendra Prakashan Trust, 2013 (5).

36. Calais-Germain, *Respiration, anatomie, geste respiratoire*, 203.

37. Clerc, *La Respiration contrôle du souffle, manières et art de respirer, l'art de vibrer à l'unisson du tout*, 54.

38. *Pranayama: The Science of Breathing in Mind Management*, 18.

39. Farhi, *The Breathing Book*, 144.

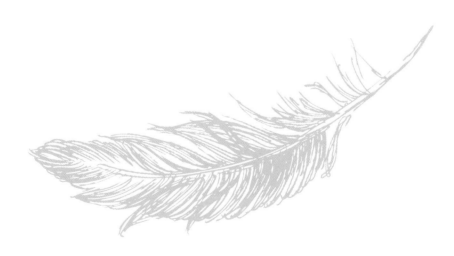

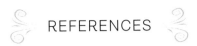

REFERENCES

De Gasquet, Bernadette. *Abdominaux: arrêtez le massacre!* Vanves, France: Marabout, 2009. English edition: *Abs: Stop the Massacre!* Seattle: Amazon Digital Services, 2013.

The Hatha Yoga Pradipika. Translated by Brian Dana Akers. YogaVidya.com, 2002.

Upanishads. Translated by Friedrich Max Müller. New York: Dover Publications, 1962.

The Yoga Sutras of Patañjali. Translated by Edwin F. Bryant. New York: North Point Press, 2009.

See also: books, articles, lectures, and works of Dr. Florence Villien, Daniel Kieffer, and Tony Courthiade

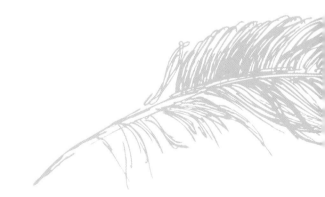

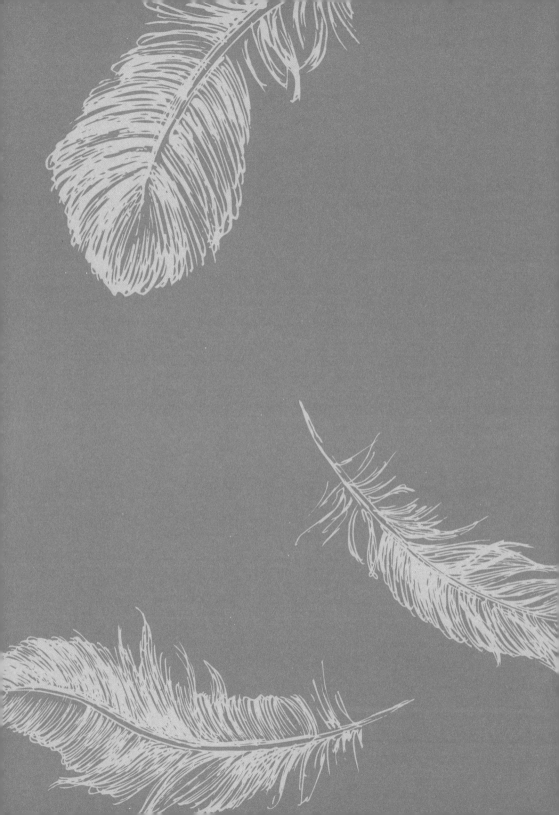

ACKNOWLEDGMENTS

I'm immensely grateful to my yoga instructors for their teachings, and to EFY and FNEY* for the wealth of knowledge and wellness practices in which they immerse their students and members.

I'm thinking of my main instructor, Jean-Pierre Laffez, in particular, and of Andrée Maman, both of whom were always available to answer any questions I had and had an active role in this work.

Warm thanks to the cardiologist Guy Taïeb, who invested his generosity, competence, and pedagogical talent in this project by reading and rereading, clarifying points that remained unclear, and improving the text overall.

Thanks to Laetitia Motard for our conversations on this subject and for her encouragement, and to Ghislaine Gasper and Catherine Ciprut for their advice.

I'm grateful to my husband, my first loyal reader, for his sharp, outside perspective. His assistance has always been precious to me. I owe to him a large part of the photos I used for the illustrations.

Finally, my gratitude goes to Laurence Auger, of Éditions La Plage, for her trust.

* EFY, École Française de Yoga (French Yoga School), is affiliated with FNEY, the Fédération Nationale des Enseignants de Yoga (The National Federation of Yoga Instructors).

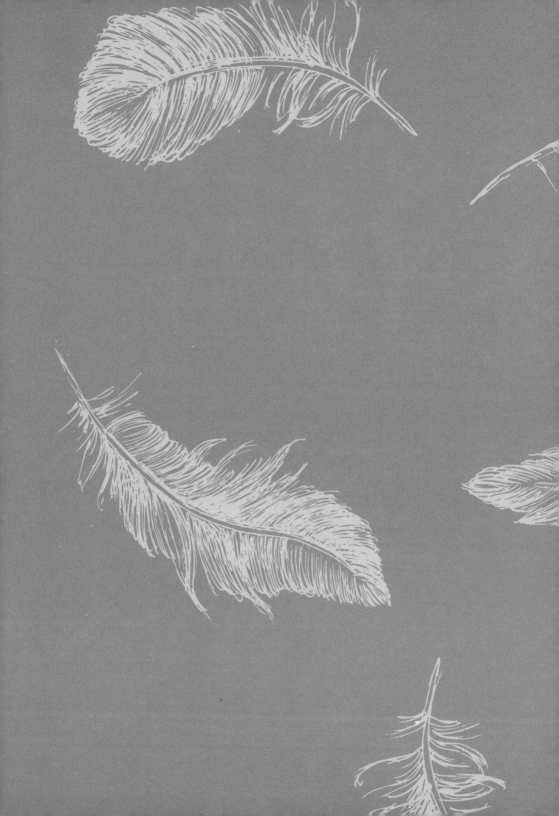

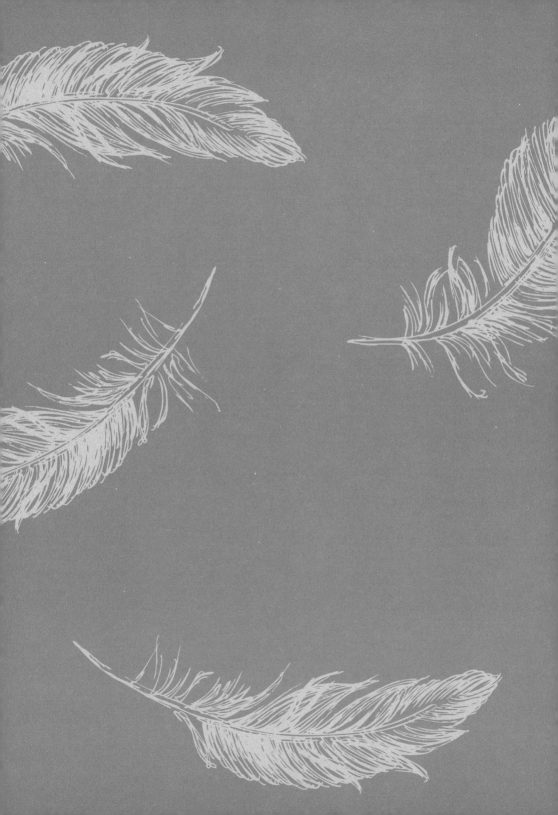

About the Author

YAEL BLOCH initially discovered yoga seeking relief from back pain. A former engineer, she began training as a yoga teacher in New York in 2001 and completed her training at the École Française de Yoga in Paris. She has three children and lives in Bucharest, where she teaches yoga and meditation classes. She is a regular contributor to the French yoga journal *Les Carnets du Yoga*.